I0071693

WHAT IN THE WORLD IS ANGIOPLASTY?

WHAT IN THE WORLD IS
ANGIOPLASTY?

Dr. Austin Mardon · Sabika Sami · Maha Saleem
Hafsa Saleem · Katie Tulloch · Madeline Langier
Lea Touliopoulos · Karanveer Kaushal
Kibrom Makaby · Khushi Shah · Madeleine Landell
Lydia Sochan · Laura Orsini

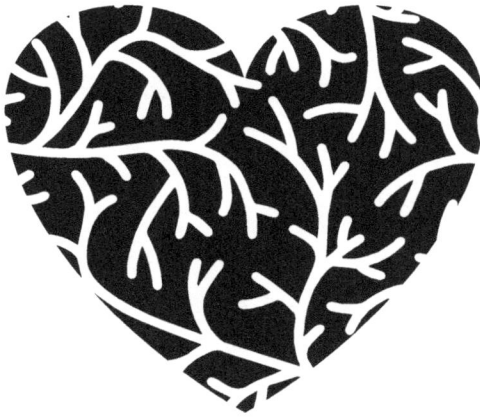

GM PRESS 2021

Copyright © 2021 by Austin Mardon, Sabika Sami, Maha Saleem, Hafsa Saleem, Katie Tulloch, Madeline Langier, Lea Touliopoulos, Karanveer Kaushal, Kibrom Makaby, Khushi Shah, Madeleine Landell, Lydia Sochan, & Laura Orsini.

All rights reserved. This book or any portion thereof may not be reproduced or used in any manner whatsoever without the express written permission of the publisher except for the use of brief quotations in a book review or scholarly journal.

First Printing: 2021

Typeset, Cover Design & Illustrations by Coralie Larochelle

ISBN 978-1-77369-246-3

Golden Meteorite Press
103 11919 82 St NW
Edmonton, AB T5B 2W3
www.goldenmeteoritepress.com

CONTENTS

SABIKA SAMI
INTRODUCTION

At the dawn of the 20th century, cardiovascular disease (CVD) was responsible for 10% of all deaths worldwide (Gaziano, 2006). Still, since 2001 that figure had grown to 30% and became the leading cause of death worldwide (Gaziano, 2006). In aid of technological advances, angioplasty has been used to treat a variety of cardiovascular diseases such as peripheral arterial disease (PAD), critical limb ischemia (CLI), coronary heart disease (CHD), and thrombosis (Gaziano, 2006). All of these cardiovascular diseases involve a build-up of plaque in the arteries (Gaziano, 2006). Angioplasty, more recently being referred to as PCI (percutaneous coronary intervention), is a treatment for cardiovascular disease and is often associated with being a quick and minimally invasive procedure often used as an alternative to coronary bypass surgery (McDermott, 2008). Angioplasty has its positives as it is suitable for establishing a quick and easy method to relieve the body's tissues from denaturing from a lack of blood, along with the pro that it is not time-consuming nor is it as risky as other surgeries; however, there are risks of bleeding and puncture site complications which is seen in 2% to 4% of angioplasties (McDermott, 2008). All risks can be exemplified by hypertension, obesity, heparin and the use of large catheters (McDermott, 2008). In any case, though, individuals who suffer from myocardial infarction, more commonly known as a heart attack, have a buildup of a fatty substance called plaque throughout the arteries, which has a multitude of factors such as reducing or completely stopping blood flow or the formation of a blood clot (Spiliopoulos, 2019). The prime purpose of angioplasty is to elevate all symptoms of plaque build-up from reoccurring again (Spiliopoulos, 2019). During the angioplasty procedure, cardiologists use a thin and long catheter to be guided through arterial tubes towards the blockage site. The catheter itself consists of a balloon that inflates to provide room for a stent- a small mesh tube to be placed to support the arteries wall to keep it open (Spiliopoulos, 2019). The catheter is then removed, and the

stent remains in the body; the whole operation requires minimum healing time and speedy recovery (Spiliopoulos, 2019). Some other rules and
techniques are utilized in angioplasty, often overlapping with multitudes
of different areas of studies, which shall be discussed further. The chapters
beyond the introduction will explore what angioplasty is, how it works,
and its significance in our society today and in the future. Finally, it will
discuss people's general health and well-being in industrialized nations
compared with the ever-advancing scientific world.

A BACKGROUND ON ANGIOPLASTY

The cardiovascular system is one of the most intricate and fascinating structures of the human body (Pugsley et al., 2000). With the heart at its core and an extensive network of blood vessels spread throughout the body, the cardiovascular system effectively distributes blood, delivers essential nutrients, and removes waste products from every single cell in the body (Pugsley et al., 2000). In addition, it plays a fundamental role in maintaining the homeostasis and proper functioning of all other bodily systems (Pugsley et al., 2000). Consequently, any complications within the cardiovascular system can have severe negative impacts on other parts of the body, taking a toll on one's overall health (World Health Organization, 2017). As reported by the World Health Organization, cardiovascular disease is the leading cause of death globally (World Health Organization, 2017). Research in cardiovascular diseases has been on the rise for the past few decades, with a focus on prevention and treatment mechanisms. One of the most revolutionary discoveries in the area was angioplasty in 1964 (Payne, 2001). Angioplasty is a non-surgical and non-invasive intervention used to restore narrowed blood vessels in the body (Chhabra, 2020). This chapter will discuss a brief overview of the biology of the cardiovascular system and cardiovascular disease and then delve into the historical development of angioplasty and its mechanisms.

The cardiovascular system comprises three main components: the heart, blood vessels, and blood (Pugsley et al., 2000). Blood vessels are of three types: arteries take blood out of the heart, veins bring blood back to the heart, and capillaries are a tiny network of vessels that connect veins and arteries while surfacing every cell in the body (Pugsley et al., 2000). The heart contains four chambers: the right atrium, left atrium, right ventricle, and left ventricle (Pugsley et al., 2000). Blood is collected in the atriums and pumped back out through the ventricles (Pugsley et al., 2000). There are two circulation pathways: pulmonary and systemic (Pugsley et al., 2000).

Pulmonary circulation carries blood from the heart to the lungs, releasing carbon dioxide and replenishing its oxygen supply (Pugsley et al., 2000). It leaves via the pulmonary artery from the right ventricle and enters the heart via the pulmonary vein to the left atrium (Pugsley et al., 2000). Systemic circulation then carries the blood from the heart to the rest of the body (Pugsley et al., 2000). It leaves via the aorta from the left ventricle, goes to the capillaries where oxygen and carbon dioxide exchange occurs, and then enters the veins and returns to the right atrium via the superior and inferior vena cava (Pugsley et al., 2000). Replenishing trillions of cells with oxygen in a matter of milliseconds is genuinely remarkable and crucial to human existence (Pugsley et al., 2000). This process occurs continuously, on a timed basis, from when an individual is born until the moment they die (Pugsley et al., 2000). Oxygen is used in cellular respiration, which provides energy to the cell, allowing for proper function (Pugsley et al., 2000). The cardiovascular system also plays a collaborative and pivotal role in the tasks of other bodily systems, including the digestive system, lymphatic system and respiratory system (Pugsley et al., 2000).

Cardiovascular diseases are disorders pertaining to the heart and blood vessels, including coronary artery diseases, cerebrovascular disease, peripheral vascular disease, rheumatic heart disease, congenital heart disease, deep vein thrombosis and pulmonary embolism (World Health Organization, 2017). A common cause for many of these diseases is the narrowing or blockage of the veins or arteries, known as thrombosis, preventing adequate circulation throughout the body (Coronary Artery Disease, n.d.). Blood vessels are lined on the inside with a protective layer of cells, known as the endothelium, which is smooth and elastic (Coronary Artery Disease, n.d.). Blockage of blood vessels occurs due to the build-up of cholesterol or fatty deposits in the vessel walls, also known as plaques (Coronary Artery Disease, n.d.). A solid cap forms on the outside of the plaque and the soft fatty deposits remain inside (Coronary Artery Disease, n.d.). Over time, platelets start to form around the plaque, creating clots (Coronary Artery Disease, n.d.). They can damage the endothelium and its elastic function, causing it to narrow (Coronary Artery Disease, n.d.). Blood clots may even break off from the origin and travel through the blood to other parts of the body, impacting the circulation elsewhere (Coronary

Artery Disease, n.d.). Narrowing of the blood vessels can also occur due to high sugar levels, infection, blood vessel defects from birth, or blood vessel spasms in which they narrow in response to certain factors, like stress (Bhimji & Cunha, 2019). Moreover, arteritis is a condition that causes the narrowing of arteries due to inflammation (Bhimji & Cunha, 2019).

In essence, the damage of blood vessels through narrowing and blockage is quite problematic. It forms an obstacle for regular circulation in the body, leading to various cardiovascular diseases. Atherosclerosis, which directly translates to a state of the hardening of the arteries, occurs from blood clotting inside the arteries (Bhimji & Cunha, 2019). When this occurs in the heart's arteries, it is known as coronary artery disease and can lead to chest pain or even a heart attack (World Health Organization, 2017). In cerebrovascular disease, adequate blood is not supplied to the brain because of atherosclerosis in the arteries of the brain (Bhimji & Cunha, 2019). This can result in a stroke (World Health Organization, 2017). In peripheral vascular disease, there is reduced circulation to any part of the body aside from the heart or brain due to a blocked or narrowed blood vessel (Bhimji & Cunha, 2019). Restoring blood vessels is thus an essential medical intervention that needs to be widely established and available.

Prior to the 20th century, the most common causes of death worldwide were infectious diseases and malnutrition (Gaziano, 2006). However, as the world entered an era of rapid technological development, the causes of illness and mortality took a shift (Gaziano, 2006). With improved healthcare services, nutrition, and global immunization, the burden of infectious diseases was reduced and replaced by non-infectious diseases, including cardiovascular disease (Gaziano, 2006). These are largely influenced by the impacts of industrialization, including a rise in obesity rates, physical inactivity, and the widespread use of tobacco and similar drugs (Gaziano, 2006). This epidemiological transition is observed as a country becomes more developed and transitions from low-income to middle-income and high-income (Gaziano, 2006). It is strongly correlated with changes in personal and collective wealth, social structure, and demographics (Gaziano, 2006). Cardiovascular disease became the leading cause of death in the developed world by the mid-1900s, and in the developing world by 2001 (Gaziano, 2006). It has had major social and economic impacts. In 2003 alone, the United States was estimated to spend $305 billion on cardiovascular diseases' direct and indirect costs (Gaziano, 2006). Both the high mortality and burden of these diseases had encouraged the medical community to research and investigate effective preventative and treatment measures (Gaziano, 2006). In the mid-1900s, this was particularly an important area of focus, and many renowned scientists were hard at work, including Charles Dotter.

Charles Dotter, also known as the father of interventional radiology, is accredited with the discovery of angioplasty (Payne, 2001). Dotter was born on June 14, 1920, in Boston, Massachusetts (Payne, 2001). As a child, he was very curious, intelligent, and always filled with energy (Payne, 2001). He had a keen interest in working with tools (Payne, 2001). Whenever he encountered a machine, he would break it apart to see how it worked, and use its parts to create new things (Payne, 2001). In 1941, Dotter completed his bachelor of arts degree from Duke University (Payne, 2001). Following this, he attended medical school at Cornell University; after his residency, he was offered a full-time faculty member position there (Payne, 2001). In 1952, he was offered a chairman position for the Department of Radiology at the University of Oregon Medical School, becoming the youngest person to hold such a position in the country (Payne, 2001). Dotter had a keen interest in angiocardiography and interventional radiology and published over 300 papers in these disciplines throughout his career (Payne, 2001).

Before Dotter discovered angioplasty, treatment for thrombosis included surgery or medications that aimed to dissolve the blood clots (Payne, 2001). Medications were not very reliable (Payne, 2001). Surgical procedures took many days, involved anesthesia, and often resulted in mortality or surgical morbidity (Payne, 2001). Before surgery could be performed, an angiogram was obtained to visualize the blockage (Payne, 2001). This was done by percutaneously injecting a catheter, which is a soft hollow tube, to release a contrast agent into the blood vessels (Payne, 2001). The contrast agent would allow for blood vessels and the surrounding areas to be highlighted in X-ray images (Payne, 2001). Multiple photos were taken simultaneously to observe the blood flow and disclose the blockage (Payne, 2001). A scalpel, need, and thread was then used to perform surgery (Payne, 2001). Dotter dreamed of developing a treatment mechanism through which the blood vessel could be treated without surgery (Payne, 2001). He even designed his own conceptual trademark with a wrench and cross pipe (Payne, 2001). This signified that if a plumber could open up and clear out pipes, then physicians should be able to do the same to blood vessels (Payne, 2001).

In 1963, Dotter performed an angiogram on a patient and accidentally dislodged the blood vessel blockage with the catheter (Payne, 2001). In his words, he "recanalized an occluded right iliac artery bypassing a percutaneously introduced catheter retrogradely through the occlusion to perform an abdominal aortogram in a patient with renal artery stenosis" (Payne, 2001). This was miraculous and sparked the idea of angioplasty. Dotter reported this finding in the Czechoslovak Radiological Congress in June, and immediately after began to investigate and further develop this treatment (Payne, 2001). On January 16th, 1964, Dotter used this treatment for the first time on 82-year-old Laura Shaw (Payne, 2001). She had an ulcer on her foot and had gangrenous toes (Payne, 2001). Many physicians recommended amputation or surgery, but she refused (Payne, 2001). Dotter inserted a catheter percutaneously and used it to dislodge the blockage (Payne, 2001). Within minutes, her foot warmed up. Within a week the pain was gone, and the ulcer healed not long after (Payne, 2001). Follow-ups with the patient proved that Dotter's technique was in fact successful (Payne, 2001). This technique went on to be called "percutaneous transluminal angioplasty" (Payne, 2001). For some time, the medical community, and particularly vascular surgeons, we're not very fond of it and preferred that catheters only be used in angiograms (Payne, 2001).

In 1974, a cardiologist from Zurich by the name of Andreas Grüntzig developed a balloon catheter that was capable of dilating peripheral arteries (Payne, 2001). This procedure employed the same technique as that of Dotter, but a deflated balloon was put over the catheter tip, and inflated once inside the blood vessel to dilate it (Barton et al., 2014). In 1978, he reported the success of percutaneous transluminal angioplasty in an article in the *Lancet*, attracting the attention of many physicians (Payne, 2001). Together, he and Dotter fought the criticism and by 1981, percutaneous angioplasty had been widely accepted (Payne, 2001).

In the coming decades, these procedures were further developed and applied (Iqbal et al., 2013). Although balloon angioplasty revolutionized the treatment of cardiovascular disease, it came with a few obstacles (Iqbal et al., 2013). First, elastic recoil often occurred within blood vessels, causing re-narrowing after angioplasty (Iqbal et al., 2013). This was found to occur almost immediately in 5-10% of patients, resulting in an urgent need for surgery (Iqbal et al., 2013). In addition, sometimes the angioplasty induced tearing of the endothelial cells, which led to platelet aggregation and blood vessel blockage once again (Iqbal et al., 2013). The balloon also induced muscle cell necrosis, ensuing proliferation and migration of medial smooth muscle cells into the region (Iqbal et al., 2013). This could cause neointimal restenosis, which is the inflammation of blood vessel walls due to proliferation and migration of cells (Iqbal et al., 2013). These reasons compromised the outcome of balloon angioplasty and led to further development of the treatment (Iqbal et al., 2013).

To combat these issues, bare-metal stents were introduced to the device (Iqbal et al., 2013). A bare-metal stent is a stainless steel wire-mesh structure that is mounted over the balloon catheter (Iqbal et al., 2013). It expands with the balloon and scaffolds the blood vessel upon dilation (Iqbal et al., 2013). In 1985, Julio César Palmaz and his colleagues were the first to implant this stent into an artery (Iqbal et al., 2013). Some modifications were made to this by another scientist named Schatz, and thus, the Palmaz-Schatz stent was brought to the market in 1987 (Iqbal et al., 2013). However, this device did have some drawbacks. The stents had high metallic density, were bulky, and resulted in in-stent restenosis - which is the formation of blood clots on coronary stents (Iqbal et al., 2013). To combat this issue, drug-eluting stents were introduced (Iqbal et al., 2013). The regular metal stents were coated with antiproliferative drugs, immunosuppressive drugs, and drugs that inhibit cell migration (Iqbal et al., 2013). These drugs were incorporated into a polymer before being applied to the metal stent and were released slowly over a few weeks following angioplasty (Iqbal et al., 2013). In 2006, it was found that drug-eluting stents introduced other risks (Iqbal et al., 2013). A new antiplatelet agent was discovered, which combined aspirin and clopidogrel (Iqbal et al., 2013). This significantly reduced prior issues with the procedure (Iqbal et al., 2013). Both drug-eluting stents and bare-metal stents were used in angioplasty procedures depending on the circumstances (Iqbal et al., 2013).

Over the next few years, there were multiple refinements made to the materials and design of these devices (Iqbal et al., 2013). Cobalt-chromium alloys replaced stainless steel in the metal stents, allowing them to be thinner (Iqbal et al., 2013). Recently, these have been replaced with platinum-chromium alloys, making them have high radiopacity, strength, and conformation (Iqbal et al., 2013). Better polymers and anti-retinoic drugs have been incorporated in the drug-eluting stents, including everolimus and paclitaxel (Iqbal et al., 2013). The balloons used in angioplasty have also been refined to treat blood vessels with very small diameters (Iqbal et al., 2013).

The general theories regarding percutaneous transluminal angioplasty were applied more broadly and refined to develop treatments for various cardiovascular diseases. Some examples include coronary artery stent angioplasty which is done in the coronary artery, cerebral angioplasty which is done in the brain, or carotid angioplasty which is done in the neck. Another type of angioplasty, which was more recently developed, is laser angioplasty (Stanek, 2019). This employs the use of a laser light, a connector that directs the laser light, a laser catheter with optical fibres, and the catheter tip from where the laser energy transmits into the blood vessel (Stanek, 2019). The laser light is able to destroy the plaque buildup and clear the blood vessel (Stanek, 2019). Some advantages of it include smoother passage and no in-stent restenosis (Stanek, 2019). A drawback is that laser catheters cannot create sufficiently wide channels in the blood vessels, and so a balloon dilation may still be required (Stanek, 2019).

Nonetheless, the discovery of angioplasty was truly ground-breaking and has saved countless lives to date. It is a procedure that has revolutionized medical care for cardiovascular disease and continues to be developed and evolved to maximize effectiveness.

PROMINENT CONTRIBUTIONS TO ANGIOPLASTY DEVELOPMENT

The use of angioplasty to treat patients with cardiovascular disease has been one of the most revolutionary medical achievements of the 20th century. It was accomplished through the hard work and innovative research of a number of prominent scientists. To further understand the progression of that research and how it played out, it is crucial to delve into the lives and studies of these prominent figures.

Right before the turn of the century, Carl Weigert was the first to lay the foundations of research into treatment methods for myocardial infarction, also known as a heart attack (Smilowitz & Feit, 2016). Ironically, he was the cousin of Paul Erlich, who played a similar role in laying the foundation in the study of immunology (Morrison, 1924). Weigert was born on March 19th, 1845 in Münsterberg, Germany (Morrison, 1924). He lived a relatively simple life and his parents owned an inn (Morrison, 1924). Nonetheless, he was a keen student and went on to study medicine in the universities of Breslau and Berlin in 1862 (Morrison, 1924). There, he studied under a number of notable scientists, including Rudolf Heidenhain, Rudolf Virchow, Wilhelm Waldeyer and Julius Cohnheim (Morrison, 1924). Early on in his career, he conducted revolutionary research regarding smallpox (Morrison, 1924). A smallpox epidemic had broken out in Breslau, and he used this opportunity to study the bacteria in smallpox (Morrison, 1924). In 1971, he published a paper regarding his work, which was the first-ever use of staining bacteria as a diagnostic method to examine pathological tissue (Dunham & Herter, 1907). He went on to do considerable research in the field of pathology, including in the pathogenesis of tuberculosis and coagulation necrosis (Morrison, 1924). In particular, he made a number of notable contributions to the area of coagulation necrosis, which was introduced to him by his former teacher, Julius Cohnheim (Morrison, 1924). Coagulation necrosis involves cell death, caused by a lack of blood flow, and occurs following an episode of myocardial infarction (Morrison,

1924). Through his research, Weigert connected that myocardial infarction resulted from the obstruction of coronary arterioles, which could thereby lead to coagulation necrosis (Morrison, 1924). In 1880, he published a paper in Germany titled "Ueber die pathologischen Gerinnungsvorgänge" which translates to "About the pathological coagulation processes" (Weigert, 1880). In this paper, he was the first to draw this connection between myocardial infarction and coronary occlusion (Weigert, 1880). Although he tends to receive little acknowledgement for his contributions to medicine and pathology, he was able to lay the framework for what was yet to come in the understanding of myocardial infarction.

Around 30 years later, the field of cardiology saw another revolutionary scientist, this time in America - James Herrick. James Herrick was born on August 11, 1861, in Illinois (Olszewski, 2018). Prior to his medical career, he led a very regular life. He studied literature at the University of Michigan and became a high school teacher, teaching subjects like Latin, Greek and History (Olszewski, 2018). However, during this time, he became passionate about medicine and decided to enroll in medical studies at Rush Medical College in Chicago (Olszewski, 2018). He graduated with his MD in 1888 (Olszewski, 2018). While pursuing his medical career, he conducted medical research and published several papers, particularly on the topic of diagnostics (Olszewski, 2018). Likewise, he was particularly interested in studying the diseases of the heart and focused his research extensively on this topic (Olszewski, 2018). One particular study that defined his career as a diagnostician, was a report on myocardial infarction, which he published in 1912 (Olszewski, 2018). In this report, he became the first American physician to introduce a clinicopathological description of myocardial infarction (Olszewski, 2018). In his paper, he linked myocardial infarction to coronary occlusion like Weigert had (Herrick, 1912). Likewise, he hypothesized that coronary thrombosis - which refers to the formation of blood clots in the arteries-was the direct cause of necrosis in the heart tissues and, subsequently, for myocardial infarction (Smilowitz & Feit, 2016). Moreover, he was amongst the first to voice the perspective that a coronary thrombosis could be treated and a myocardial infarction did not necessarily need to be fatal (Olszewski, 2018). Although Herrick himself is accredited to have given importance to absolute bed rest following a myocardial infarction, his novel perspective gave rise to research into several innovative and optimistic treatment methods (Olszewski, 2018). However, researchers differed in their understanding of coronary thrombosis, and many saw it as a result of myocardial infarction as opposed to its cause (Smilowitz & Feit, 2016). As a result, the search for treatment methods over the next century was slow (Smilowitz & Feit, 2016).

The first therapy method for myocardial infarction was thrombolytic - medications that could break down blood clots. These were game-changer in the field of cardiology at the time. In 1933, Dr. William Smith Tillet, who was an Associate Professor of Medicine and Director of the Biological Division at Johns Hopkins University conducted research regarding a thrombolytic agent (Tillett & Garner, 1933). This thrombolytic agent was streptokinase, a fibrinolysin produced by hemolytic streptococci bacteria (Tillett & Garner, 1933). He successfully isolated the streptokinase in stable form for use (Tillett & Garner, 1933). In 1947, Dr. Sol Sherry, who was a student of Tillet, worked alongside him to investigate the therapeutic potential of streptokinase (Sikri & Bardia, 2007). In 1950, he became the first to use streptokinase for thrombolytic therapy for cardiovascular disease (Sikri & Bardia, 2007). However, thrombolytics were primarily ignored over the next 30 years due to the uncertainty regarding the etiology of myocardial infarction and whether coronary thrombosis was a cause or a result of it (Smilowitz & Feit, 2016). It wasn't until 1980 that enough research could prove the reliability of thrombolytic agents. In 1980, the National Institutes of Health provided guidelines for the use of thrombolytic therapy (Smilowitz & Feit, 2016). Nonetheless, there were still several limitations in thrombolytic therapy. For instance, it failed to achieve adequate coronary reperfusion in at least a third of cases. It was associated with high rates of hemorrhagic stroke in patients above 75 years of age (Smilowitz & Feit, 2016). Likewise, even following thrombolytic therapy, patients were still at for coronary re-occlusion (Smilowitz & Feit, 2016). This demonstrated the dire need for a new and more effective treatment method.

This new treatment method came at the hands of American radiologist Charles Theodore Dotter. He is known as the "father of intervention" to develop the medical specialty of interventional radiology (Payne, 2001). As described in the previous chapter, he first described coronary angioplasty through his work in this discipline (Iqbal et al., 2013). His marvellous discovery of angioplasty was quite marvellous and took place in 1963 when he accidentally dislodged a patient's coronary occlusion while performing an angiogram (Payne, 2001). Through this event, he discovered that catheter therapy could be used to treat coronary occlusion (Payne, 2021). Less than a year later, he officially performed this procedure on 82-year-old Laura Shaw on January 16th, 1964, alongside his colleague Melvin Judkins (Payne, 2001). Thus, this procedure came to be known as percutaneous transluminal angioplasty (Payne, 2001).

Dotter's discovery was genuinely revolutionary, yet it was very new to most physicians and surgeons, unsure its reliability. Later in 1964, a surgeon sent Dotter his patient, Harry Bourne, for an angiogram before the surgery he was planning to conduct (Payne, 2001). On the angiogram request form, he wrote to Dotter, "visualize but do not try to fix" (Payne, 2001). He did this to ensure that Dotter would not attempt to carry out the catheter procedure he had carried out on Laura Shaw just a few months prior (Payne, 2001). This was due to a lack of trust in both him and the procedure itself. Dotter, however, being very confident and faithful in his procedure, went forth with it (Payne, 2001). In particular, as Dotter observed through the angiogram, Bourne had two arteries in which narrowing could be observed: his superficial femoral artery and his deep femoral artery (Payne, 2001). Dotter decided to perform his procedure in Bourne's deep femoral artery, which he later mentioned only took him "a moment" to do (Payne, 2001). For the superficial femoral artery, the original surgical procedure the surgeon had planned was carried out (Payne, 2001). Dotter continued to meticulously observe and follow up with this patient for the next couple of years and actually formed quite a friendship with him (Payne, 2001). After about a year following the procedure, the two took a hike up 11,000 feet on Mt. Hood - this was quite revolutionary and demonstrated the success of his procedure in returning the patient to regular health (Payne, 2001). Eventually, the surgical treatment conducted on the superficial femoral artery failed; however, the deep femoral artery was well intact even five years following the procedure (Payne, 2001).

This demonstrated just how revolutionary Dotter's discovery was. However, this was yet to be realized by the physicians and surgeons of the time. Dotter had demonstrated that this procedure could be performed in the leg arteries, which are much larger and less risky than coronary arteries (Payne, 2001). Nevertheless, physicians were cautious about accepting this procedure, never mind extending it to the coronary arteries (Payne, 2001). Part of this had to do with Dotter's ignorance towards social norms and medical establishments (Payne, 2001). He was very innovative and passionate about new ideas and was sometimes called "Crazy Charlie" because many physicians around him couldn't understand his ideas (Payne, 2001). However, Dotter's discovery was quite impressed by the German cardiologist Andrea Gruntzig (Payne, 2001). In contrast to Dotter, Gruntzig was a well-respected and disciplined figure in the medical community (Payne, 2001). As Judkins, the former colleague of Dotter who had assisted him in first performing his procedure, said regarding the two, "Dr. Dotter frequently presents ideas in a nonconservative way. Now Dr. Grüntzig is just the opposite; he presents himself as super-cautious, where Charlie presents himself as aggressive" (Payne, 2001). With that level of respect and acceptance, Gruntzig was able to develop further the procedure that Dotter had laid the foundations for. While Dotter was the first to officially implement the use of percutaneous transluminal angioplasty and describe its further implications in coronary arteries, Gruntzig became the first to use it in coronary arteries over a decade later (Iqbal et al., 2013).

Andreas Gruntzig was born on June 25, 1939 in Dresden Germany (Barton et al., 2014). Having been born just shortly before World War II and losing his father at a young age, Gruntzig did not have an easy childhood (Barton et al., 2014). However, education was always prioritized by his mother and he was able to get a decent education (Barton et al., 2014). Having graduated with the highest honours, he decided to attain his medical degree at the University of Heidelberg and graduated with it in 1964 (Barton et al., 2014). Gruntzig went on to conduct research in the area of epidemiology before transitioning to clinical research (Barton et al., 2014). In 1969, he became a clinical fellow at the Max Ratschow Clinic, an angiology clinic in Darmstadt, Germany (Barton et al., 2014). While working at this clinic, a patient asked Gruntzig whether it was possible to "clean" arteries like one could clean a pipe instead of using drugs or surgery (Barton et al., 2014). Gruntzig was intrigued by this idea and later recounted that he found it "fascinating" (Barton et al., 2014). Around this time, he happened to attend a lecture at the Frankfurt Vascular Medicine Circle, where Dr. Eberhard Zeitler discussed his experience using the novel Dotter method (Barton et al., 2014). Gruntzig was impressed and surprised that such a method existed to "clean" arteries like his patient had asked him just a short while earlier (Barton et al., 2014). He visited Zeitler to understand further Dotter's technique (Barton et al., 2014). He eventually moved to the University of Zurich in Switzerland and invited Zeitler to teach his method there (Barton et al., 2014). After learning the technique, Gruntzig began performing percutaneous transluminal angioplasties in 1971 (Barton et al., 2014).

During his time in Zurich, the idea for the balloon catheter was introduced (Barton et al., 2014). Due to a general lack of support, it took Gruntzig 2 years to get access to functional balloon catheters for use (Barton et al., 2014). On February 12, 1974, Gruntzig was able to perform the first-ever procedure using the balloon catheter (Barton et al., 2014). Shortly after, Grunzig developed the double-lumen balloon catheter and demonstrated its use in a patient in 1975 (Barton et al., 2014). His success led him to shift towards looking for a solution to coronary arteries - to do so; he began experimenting with catheters of reduced diameter (Barton et al., 2014). He was eventually able to come up with a feasible design and presented it at the Deutsche Gesellschaft für Kreislaufforschung in Germany and at the American Heart Association's Scientific Sessions in Miami, which both took place in 1976 (Barton et al., 2014). On May 9th, 1977, with the assistance of Dr. Richard K. Myler, Gruntzig took on the difficult challenge of performing a percutaneous transluminal angioplasty in the coronary artery of a patient in San Francisco (Barton et al., 2014). This procedure was successful and was a milestone in interventional cardiology (Iqbal et al., 2013). Only four months later, in September of 1977, Gruntzig performed the same procedure inpatient while he was conscious (Iqbal et al., 2013). He carried out 60 percutaneous transluminal coronary angioplasties (PTCA) by April of 1979 (Barton et al., 2014). His work became widely recognized, and he became known as one of the fathers of modern interventional cardiology (Smilowitz & Feit, 2016).

Following Gruntzig's demonstration of the PTCA technique, American cardiologist Geoffrey Hartzler introduced this technique as a treatment method for acute myocardial infarction (Smilowitz & Feit, 2016). He performed the first PTCA on a myocardial infarction patient (Smilowitz & Feit, 2016). This became one of the only treatment methods for myocardial infarction aside from thrombolytic therapy (Smilowitz & Feit, 2016). However, many were skeptical about whether this treatment method was more effective than thrombolytic therapy (Smilowitz & Feit, 2016). Initially, a number of studies showed that there was no real improvement in terms of effectiveness (Smilowitz & Feit, 2016). However, eventually, it was deemed as a much more effective treatment solution (Smilowitz & Feit, 2016). A paper published in 2003, a meta-analysis of randomized control trials looking at the comparison between PTCA and thrombolytic therapy, found that PTCA reduced early mortality, reinfarction, and stroke (Keeley et al., 2003).

As research progressed in the field in the next few years, there was a new addition to it, stents. However, it was none other than Dotter who had also introduced the use of stents back in 1964, as a method to improve the stability of the diseased arterial wall (Smilowitz & Feit, 2016). In 1986, Dr. Jacques Puel, from Toulouse, France, became the first to use a stent on March 26, 1986 (Smilowitz & Feit, 2016). He was followed by Dr. Ulrich Sigwart, from Lausanne, Switzerland on June 12, 1986 (Smilowitz & Feit, 2016). The use of stents in treatment methods was truly revolutionary. A few years following them, in 1991, Dr. Gary Roubin became the first to use coronary stenting in the treatment for acute myocardial infarction (Iqbal et al., 2013).

Metal stents, however, didn't come without limitation. In particular, in-stent restenosis would occur, which refers to the narrowing of blood vessels at the site of the stent (Smilowitz & Feit, 2016). Researchers began looking for solutions to combat this and make stents more effective overall. In 2001, Dr. Eduardo Sousa of Sao Paulo, Brazil, discovered the first drug-eluting stent (Sousa et al., 2001). This drug was called sirolimus and could essentially be coated onto the stent and prevent the growth of scar tissue on the artery lining (Sousa et al., 2001). This discovery was truly remarkable and further progressed the use of stents in myocardial infarction treatment.

Over the next few years, the FDA approved a number of other stents for use in treatments (Iqbal et al., 2013). Likewise, percutaneous transluminal coronary angioplasty has become a widely used procedure, alongside the addition of stents and drug-eluting stents. None of this would be possible without the crucial contributions of the notable figures discussed in this chapter. With their contributions, this treatment method has saved thousands of lives and will no doubt continue to do so in the future.

THE SIGNIFICANCE OF ANGIOPLASTY

In the history of the human race, key inventions, innovations and ideas have opened doors to great leaps in the quality of life people experience. The understanding of one process or phenomenon leads to the discovery of many other interrelated topics. Examples of this include the invention of the wheel, running water, and even the evolution of the community among humans. Metalworking could not have been established without the discovery of fire and its interaction with the ores themselves. Modern advancements have largely been technologically based and in scientific areas such as chemistry, physics and imaging, communications, transmission and utilization of energy, material synthesis, and nanotechnology. Beyar (2013) attributes modern bursts of advancements in the medical field to "our understanding of the molecular mechanisms of disease, along with the ability to design complex molecules." The invention of angioplasty was one of these key advancements in the medical field and has been one that has had a large wave of effect on many areas of life and treatment. Not only has it enabled significant technological and medical innovations, but it has also had a profound impact on the lives of the patients that undergo the procedure to improve their health.

An illness or disease can have a devastating effect on the quality of life of an individual because of the disease's primary symptoms and the secondary social and functional consequences and complications that result from having ongoing health issues. Symptoms of commonly treated illnesses we will be discussing that are treated using angioplasty-related methods include swelling, resting or active pain, kidney failure, stroke, wounds that do not heal, gangrene, and even limb amputation. The secondary effects they have on the social and economic lives of patients are also deeply affecting because their symptoms can affect their ability to work, socialize with those around them, or keep up with the activities of daily living that contribute to their overall health. In countries like Canada, the expenses of medical bills are not one that will debilitate a family or individual as much as it would in a country such as the United States. Insurance and legislation around universal health care ensure a least a little stability in the expectations to pay that are put upon the individual receiving care, but that does not mean that a person is still able to work their job or their regular hours when receiving potentially life-saving treatments. The expenses of everyday life can pile up in the form of bills and loan payments, especially if the individual has any dependents. The social impacts from experiencing a debilitating illness can be widespread too, depending on who the individual is and what they enjoy doing. Large changes in a person's social life or ability to perform their normal tasks can trigger mental health problems too, including depression, anxiety, or social anxiety, all of which have cascading effects on their physical health, ability to work and play, and their financial health.

During this chapter, we will discuss several common illnesses that the human body is plagued with, but that can be treated commonly with angioplasty. As we cover these ailments, we will also study their efficacy from peer-reviewed sources, journal articles and reviews. The treatment of these illnesses has seen advancements in the efficacy and efficiency of angioplasty and its involvement with therapeutic interventions. Because angioplasty involves the vascular system that supplies all areas of the body with blood and important molecules, its use can be seen in treating diseases all over the body from the heart all the way out to limbs and appendages.

Peripheral arterial disease is an illness that is commonly treated by angioplasty, as it involves atherosclerosis - the narrowing of arteries, specifically those that supply blood mainly to the legs but also to the stomach, arms, and head. It has a high prevalence worldwide, "20% for patients over 70 years of age," with "more than 20 million adults in Europe [that] have peripheral arterial disease (PAD)" (Spiliopoulos et al., 2019). According to The American Heart Association (2016), symptoms of this process are cramping and pain in the legs, hips or other affected areas, as well as the possibility of gangrene and amputation if left untreated. Bypass surgery, a procedure which addresses the occlusion of a blood vessel by redirecting blood flow around the blockage, is an option for the treatment but is falling out of popularity compared to angioplasty because "stenting does not necessitate general anesthesia, requires less procedural time than open bypass surgery, results in low complication rates and can be easily repeated" (Spiliopoulos et al., 2019). This, however, was not the case in the early days of angioplasty and stenting when the method was being introduced and refined. An artery dilated by angioplasty at this time would close abruptly in 10% of the cases it was used, and among these patients, 30% would die (Beyar, 2013). The earliest days of treating peripheral arterial disease with angioplasty were bleak, to say the least. Beyar (2013), in a review of the cardiovascular innovations of the past, reports that restenosis within three months of the procedure was more than 30% due to injury in the process of expanding the balloon. He also writes that as more clinicians backed by industry and engineers expanded on the emerging technology of angioplasty in the four-year period of 1994-1998, the use of stents for interventions rose from "0% to 80%" (Beyar, 2013). Another technological innovation that greatly aided the use of angioplasty was the intravascular ultrasound (IVUS) which has been identified as a valuable adjunctive tool for guiding an angioplasty procedure. Described by Loffroy et al. as "a piezoelectric transducer generating sound waves after electrical stimulation at the tip of the catheter" (2020), it is similar to the way a speaker takes the electrical energy and converts it into soundwaves that the human ear can hear. IVUS produces sound waves that register sophisticated software algorithms as different types of tissue based on their acoustic properties. Intravascular ultrasound technology has become a "mandatory adjunct tool for the best outcomes" for "increasingly complex [and] technical" endovascular procedures (Loffrey et al., 2020). As angioplasty is tested for its suitability in different situations, aspects of the procedure are modified to make it more safe depending on the circumstances.

The end-stage renal disease involves a patient's kidneys being non-functional to the point that the person must have an intervention for them to operate normally. The American Kidney Fund (2020) states that common symptoms of this condition as the kidneys begin to fail to include muscle cramping, swelling of the feet and ankles, difficulty catching one's breath, trouble sleeping, an abnormally low or high amount of urine, nausea, vomiting, lack of appetite, and itching. When kidneys stop functioning abruptly, it is referred to as acute kidney failure. Signs of this can be nosebleeds, fever, abdominal and back pain, diarrhea, rash, and vomiting. Both of these are severe medical conditions and must be treated with care by clinicians. According to the American Kidney Fund, the patient "will need dialysis or a kidney transplant to live" since there is no cure for end-stage renal disease (n.d.). Generally, the agreed-upon best course of action to keep that patient alive is hemodialysis, meaning that blood is filtered through an artificial kidney that exists outside of the body. Because the kidneys are no longer functioning properly, this treatment removes salt and waste from the blood as the patient's kidneys would have before the dysfunction. To effectively do this, oftentimes, an arteriovenous fistula (AVF) will be created. An AVF is a connection between an artery and a vein that is intentionally established as a vascular access point. These vessels get stronger and persist throughout the dialysis treatment. Eldmarany et al. cite one of the most common referrals that vascular surgeons receive as being related to the "failing of their arteriovenous fistulas" (2020). This failing results from stenosis of the vessel, meaning that the walls of an artery or vein narrow due to the buildup of plaque. Angioplasty is used to fix this stenosis issue, "generally with conventional high-pressure plain balloons accompanied by bare-metal stents," though restenosis rates are high in patients followed up with a year later and need intervention. Given the seriousness of the consequences of the arteriovenous fistula failing and disrupting the ability to filter the blood of toxins in the body, intervention must be fast, effective, and lasting. Researchers devote a considerable amount of time and energy to innovating the tools used to extend the lives of hemodialysis patients and have established drug-coated balloon angiopathy as an alternative to address the high restenosis rates.

Early stent thrombosis was a major complication in angioplasty as blood would clot, causing major complications. This would eventually be remedied "by combining full stent apposition to the vessel wall using high-pressure balloons with the use of potent antiplatelet drugs" - drug-coated balloon angioplasty, as we have touched on earlier (Beyar, 2013). Drug-coated balloons have found use in the area of reducing in-stent restenosis (ISR) of implanted stents. According to Tong et al., "worldwide, more than 400000 [femoropopliteal arterial] stents are implanted... annually, 30-40% of which will develop ISR within 2-3 years of implantation" (2020). Stenosis lesions of these implanted stents are generally different from those associated with atherosclerosis. It is caused by neointimal hyperplasia - the thickening of the vascular smooth muscle cells that narrow the luminal space of the artery. These lesions are usually long and highly calcified, presenting another complication. Repeated stenting of these areas has not produced satisfactory results, though the investigation of drug-coated balloons has revealed some promise. The drug that the balloon carries is antiproliferative in nature, meaning that it will inhibit the growth and differentiation of smooth muscle cells, therefore slowing the narrowing effect of their accumulation. In their analysis, Tong et al. identified that drug-coated balloons are preferred because of their ability to deliver the antiproliferative drug locally. Compared to regular angioplasty at follow-ups six and twelve months post-procedure, drug-coated balloon stents had a higher patency rate, meaning they are more likely not to need intervention during that time. Due to the low incidence of amputation and mortality, drug-coated balloons are relatively safe methods of combating in-stent restenosis.

Lack of blood flow to the extremities, such as in peripheral arterial disease, can cause pain during muscle use and prevent wounds on these limbs from healing. Critical limb ischemia is the serious and last stage of the peripheral arterial disease which has "exceedingly high amputation rates when prompt revascularization is not offered." It boasts "a mortality of over 50% at five years after the diagnosis" (Spiliopoulos et al., 2019). Revascularization involves establishing blood flow to the foot tissue to enable metabolic activity that will lead to the healing of the foot wound, such as an ulcer. Angioplasty has been established as a useful intervention in this case because it is able to target blocked arteries that are mostly responsible for the blood supply of the area of the foot that has the wound. This concept is called angiosome and is "a three-dimensional anatomic distribution of tissues (skin, subcutaneous tissue, tendons and fascia, muscle, and underlying bone) supplied a certain artery and drained by a certain vein" (Shehata et al., 2020). In the foot, six regions are each supplied by three major arteries. Using this knowledge to plan the path of the angioplasty procedure, Shehata et al. studied outcomes compared to a group of patients with similar foot wounds who receive angioplasty that is not based on the angiosome model. The primary thing they were measuring was the complete healing of the wound and found that "all the study sample patients showed immediate hemodynamic improvement" (Shehata et al., 2020). While 92.5% of patients achieved the primary endpoint, 70.2% of the patients saw improvement in one to two months when direct perfusion was used versus the remaining 29.8% of participants whose wound healed in a longer period of six to twelve months - all of which were in the indirect perfusion group. These findings support their hypothesis that consideration of the angiosome model of the foot tissues in which the angioplasty procedure is performed have significant effects on the healing time of non-healing and life or limb threatening wounds.

Another area of medical treatment angioplasty has seen dedicated research is in its role in atherosclerotic stenosis of the intracranial arteries. Intracranial arteries are those that are within the skull. In cases of severe stenosis in which there is 70-99% narrowing of the luminal space of the artery, patients are at high risk for recurrent stroke. In the 1980s, when angioplasty alone was first explored as a treatment instead of other forms of medical management, "immediate elastic recoil of the artery, dissection, acute vessel closure, and residual stenosis >50%" was associated. However, technical success was achieved in over 80% of patients, "the rate of stroke or death within 30 days of angioplasty varied between 4% and 40%, and restenosis rates were 24-40%" (Wabnitz & Chimowitz, 2017). More recently, as other medical management methods such as antithrombotic agents have been developed which have a much lower risk of stroke, angioplasty has fallen out of popularity for treating this particular atherosclerotic stenosis, such as in data from a trial of the Vitesse Intracranial Study for Ischemic Stroke Therapy (VISSIT) using a balloon-mounted VITESSE stent as summarized by Wabnitz and Chimowitz (2017) where it showed "an absolute increase in the rate of ischemic stroke in the territory from stenting of 25.1% at one year, and the absolute risk of ischemic and hemorrhagic stroke from stenting at one year of 33.7" (Wabnitz & Chimowitz, 2017). As these statistics are not so different from those found in the 1980s, at the moment, atherosclerosis of the intracranial arteries is more commonly being treated using medical management methods other than angioplasty.

Since its inception, angioplasty has been in the area of great innovation from "the triangle of collaborations between industry, academia, and practicing physicians" (Bayer, 2013). Bayer describes the modern history and development of angioplasty as "a virtual parade of large and small industry initiatives, attempting to improve this disruptive technology in small additive steps" (2013). From balloon inflation to drug and miniaturization, angioplasty has enabled significant changes in the treatment of various areas in the field of cardiovascular disease. Angioplasty has therefore enabled a great change in the lives of many patients, who suffered from life-threatening conditions to not only improved their health but also draw a realization of why it is essential to treat your body like a temple, so the cardiovascular disease can be prevented in the first place.

UNDERSTANDING ANGIOPLASTY— WHAT IS IT SPECIFICALLY?

Angioplasty can be simply understood as a medical procedure used to treat narrowing or collapsed veins or arteries. Further, it is a mechanism in which the core elements include a needle, balloon and occasionally a stent. A stent is a small piece of metal or plastic tubing inserted into the lumen to ensure the vein or artery is dilated. The lumen is the central cavity of a cell, and in this case, of the vein or artery. In some cases, a stent is inserted and left within the artery to ensure consistent blood flow (Barton et al., 2014). The mechanism was created to eradicate vessel narrowing veins or arteries (Holzapfel et al., 2000). As a result, plaque builds up, narrowing the veins and preventing blood flow from cholesterol, calcium and other fatty substances clustered together (Chhabra, 2020). What is notable about *angioplasty* is that it is a minimally invasive and non-surgical procedure that is as simple as a needle to the skin, crucial to the treatment of atherosclerosis, which is the technical term for plaque buildup in veins and arteries (Palasubramaniam et al., 2019, Chhabra, 2020). Moreover, angioplasty does not require an operation. Instead, the procedure is done entirely through the needle and catheter, resulting in a short recovery.

Treatment for atherosclerosis is necessary, as left untreated. The result is a lack of blood and a lack of oxygen to the afflicted region, which could be the heart, brain, or legs. The lack of oxygen will inevitably result in the death of healthy cells. For example, the restricted blood flow and oxygen to the heart is the root of chest pain typically associated with a heart attack (Chhabra, 2020). Some researchers have suggested a high-carbohydrate diet, and a sedentary lifestyle is the primary cause of atherosclerosis. However, contemporary research has found that atherosclerosis is a gradual process that typically begins in early adult life (Chhabra, 2020). Further, research has found numerous contributing factors that influence vascular plaque build-ups, such as inflammation and vascular injury (Ridker, 2002, Palasubramaniam. et al., 2019). Thus, atherosclerosis is recognized as a disorder characterized by a chronic change of the inflammatory function. Further essential markers of inflammation, the innate immune response and several cell molecules have been linked to the future occurrence of myocardial infarction and stroke in both healthy populations and among those with known coronary disease (Ridker, 2002).

When afflicted with atherosclerosis of the heart, the blood flow is barricaded from the heart—resulting in a myocardial infarction, known colloquially as a heart attack. While it is relatively well understood that myocardial infarction is a leading cause of death in the developed world (Palasubramaniam et al., 2019). Less understood is angioplasty as treatment. As mentioned, angioplasty, also known as percutaneous coronary intervention (PCI), is used primarily to widen collapsing veins and arteries (Watson et al., 2018). The first successful balloon angioplasty was performed by German physician-scientists Andreas Gruntzig (1939-1985). Gruntzig invented the balloon catheter angioplasty in the early 1970s, which, once inserted, would remedy the narrowing or collapsing arteries from within the lumen (Barton et al., 2014). The angioplasty concept was introduced over 50 years ago as the "plain old balloon angioplasty" (POBA) without stenting. In the mid-1980s, the plain balloon angioplasty was limited because of an early complication of vascular recoil property and restenosis after balloon deflation, leading to the invention of bare-metal stents (Chhabra, 2020). Although there is a potential for the balloon to damage the vessel, An angioplasty directly impacts the walls of the vein or artery with a stent or balloon (Holzapfel et al. 2000). An inflatable balloon-tipped catheter is inserted through the skin. As the balloon inflates, it presses the plaque against the arterial wall and widens the luminal diameter; thereby increasing the blood flow to the heart's muscular tissue, alleviating the chest pain (Watson et al., 2018). The pressure forces the vein and, the plague, outward thereby restoring the vessel. Henceforth, angioplasty would include a balloon-tipped needle inserted through the skin into the lumen of the vein or artery. While the procedure may be fundamental in treating atherosclerosis in the heart, it is essential to treat arteries apart from the coronary (Watson et al., 2018). Since Gruntzig, modern research has produced numerous alternatives to the first balloon angioplasty. Specifically, alternate forms of an angioplasty allow for a stent to be inserted to maintain the vein's structure. In early procedures, the bare metal stent was found to cause tangible harm as the metal was found to cause inflammation and clotting in some cases (Chhabra, 2020). Specifically, permanent metal stents have the potential to increase myofibroblast migration which is a core function in wound healing and can result in in-stent restenosis (IRS)(Chhabra, 2020). In-stent restenosis is the narrowing of the artery with the stent inside reversing the procedure. These issues, which could arise from the bare metal stent, led to the development of drug-eluting stents which use a coating of an antiproliferative drug on top of the metallic structure of the stent (Chhabra, 2020).

Angioplasty with stenting is currently the treatment of choice in patients with coronary artery disease, such as unstable angina, when the heart does not receive enough blood and oxygen. Further, angioplasty is used to treat non-ST-elevation myocardial infarction (NSTEMI) and ST-elevation myocardial infarction (STEMI), and spontaneous coronary artery perforation (Chhabra, 2020). A STEMI is a severe heart attack during which one of the major arteries responsible for supplying oxygen and nutrient-rich blood to the heart muscle is blocked. Similarly, an NSTEMI is still a heart attack; however, it is much less damaging to the heart. Moreover, when performing the angioplasty, the choice of stent depends on the patient's tolerance to dual antiplatelet therapy (DAPT) and whether they have a minimal risk of bleeding (Chhabra, 2020). *Dual antiplatelet therapy* is a treatment that aims to prevent blood clotting, which contributes to heart attacks.

As mentioned, angioplasty is the treatment of choice for acute myocardial infarction. A deeper understanding includes a breakdown of the two main methods for catheterization, which are the classical transfemoral and transradial approaches. While the trans-radial approach is not the first choice of medical practitioners, the choice of procedure does profoundly depend on the patient's characteristics and the expertise available (Chhabra, 2020). The classic procedure termed the transfemoral approach is associated with easier access. Specifically, the transfemoral approach means the catheterization occurs in the femoral artery. However, there tend to be more complications at this access site, especially in obese patients. Complications include site bleeding, hematoma, major bleeding within the body, requiring a blood transfusion. Further, the femoral artery is the only source of blood to the leg. Therefore, complications with a transfemoral approach can lead to a greater chance of ischemia (Chhabra, 2020). Ischemia is a restriction in blood supply and therefore oxygen to the tissue resulting in tissue death.

In contrast to the femoral artery, the radial artery, one of the two main arteries of the forearm, can be easily penetrated and manually compressed to control bleeding. Furthermore, there is no nerve ending near the artery; therefore, the risk of neurovascular injury is minimal (Chhabra, 2020). Thus, making the radial artery a seemingly ideal location to insert the catheter. While the trans-radial approach typically involves a lengthy procedure, raised radiation exposure and anatomical variations leading to catheterization, as well as radial artery spasm. The radial artery spasms can be managed with local injection of vasodilatory medication such as nitrates and calcium channel blockers (Chhabra, 2020). Further, vasodilatory medication is used to widen the blood vessels to control the convulsions in the radial artery. Additionally, compared to the transfemoral approach, the transradial procedure requires less hospital time and is much more cost-effective (Chhabra, 2020)

In contrast to the angioplasty used to treat myocardial infarction, a carotid artery angioplasty is a procedure used to treat cerebrovascular disease, which is the third leading cause of death in the United States (Higashida et al., 2004). Various cerebrovascular disorders affect the blood vessels and blood supply to the brain. Narrowing and blockage of the blood vessels to the brain result in less oxygen, which is vital for the brain cells to stay viable. In 2004, approximately 750 000 people died from a stroke annually in the U.S, costing an estimated $45 billion in treatment and lost productivity (Higashida et al., 2004). In the U.S in 2004, the carotid occlusive disease was responsible for approximately 25% of strokes. An individual is diagnosed with the carotid occlusive disease when plaque begins to cause the carotid artery to narrow, preventing blood flow. Relevant to the general population is that extensive population-based studies have indicated that the likelihood of carotid narrowing is approximately 0.5% after age 60. However, it increases to 10% in persons older than age 80 (Higashida et al., 2004). Especially troubling is that most cerebrovascular disease cases are asymptomatic, therefore diminishing the possibility of preventative treatment.

Before 2004, the surgical carotid endarterectomy was the accepted standard of treatment of extracranial carotid occlusive revascularization disease (Higashida et al., 2004). The purpose of the procedure remains to surgically remove the plague, blocking or narrowing the carotid artery. Further, the success of a surgical carotid endarterectomy has been confirmed by multiple, randomized, controlled trials that have demonstrated its effectiveness over other reliable forms of medical therapy. However, exciting innovations in the past several years led to the emergence of carotid artery stenting as a potential therapeutic alternative to carotid endarterectomy in treating atherosclerotic carotid artery disease (Higashida et al., 2004).

While the surgical carotid endarterectomy is an effective treatment, scientific advancements about the use of stents have presented a less invasive treatment option with a low risk of injury to the carotid and significantly fewer complications (Park & Lee, 2018). The standard procedure for carotid artery stenting is to perform the stent through the femoral artery. It is a delicate procedure requiring the surgeon to insert a catheter into the obstructed area through the femoral artery to the carotid. In most cases, the site is dilated with a 3.0-mm balloon, and the surgeon can place the stent. Afterwhich, post dilatation is recommended to give the stent a larger minimum internal luminal diameter, thus reducing the chance of artery-blocking or narrowing (Park & Lee, 2018).

While stroke prevention can be achieved by modifying vascular risk factors and using antiplatelet and anticoagulant drugs, which are drugs responsible for reducing the in patients with vessel diseases like carotid stenosis, stroke prevention can be more efficiently achieved by an intervention carotid endarterectomy or carotid angioplasty and stenting (Mal et al., 2020). An intracranial vascular disease involves the arteries within the skull or at the base, and intracranial stenosis accounts for over 20% of stroke patients who can be benefited from the revascularization of abnormal arteries or veins. In the recent past, there has been a significant advancement in intracranial angioplasty and stenting due to a better understanding of the disease and the availability of better tools and technology. At the same time, extracranial vascular disease refers to carotid collapse or blockage outside of the skull and has better-defined guidelines for disease modification and has established practice guidelines (Mal et al., 2020).

Advancements in science undoubtedly led to the incorporation of laser technology into the medical field. Initially, the phrase "laser angioplasty" described the intravascular use of lasers (light amplification by stimulated emission of radiation) and was used to draw similarities to the recognized and established procedure of balloon angioplasty (Sanborn, 1988). While balloon angioplasty successfully treats severe cases of stenoses and relatively acute, totally collapsed or obstructed vessels, one of its limitations has been treating chronic total occlusions, which are entirely plaque-filled or collapsed blood vessels. Chronic total occlusions are where the ability to cross the occlusion is difficult or impossible. In these situations, laser recanalization has been proposed as a means of crossing lesions to allow for subsequent successful balloon angioplasty (Sanborn, 1988). In other words, the laser is used to restore flow to the blood vessel. A percutaneous transluminal angioplasty is a routine procedure for the treatment of peripheral arterial disease. Percutaneous being an elaborate term indicating the angioplasty catheter will be inserted through the skin. However, it is hypothesized that more extraordinary long-term angioplasty results are noted if atherosclerotic plaques are removed rather than compressed and fractured. Hence, using a laser in modern atherosclerotic procedures to eviscerate the plague has long-lasting potential beneficial to the patient (Stanek, 2019).

Therefore, in comparison to percutaneous transluminal angioplasty, there are many advantages to a peripheral laser angioplasty. Specifically, it is an easier passage through chronic and calcified occlusions. Furthermore, according to some studies, when lasers are used, there are better short-term and medium-term results in saving limbs and managing collapsing stented vessels (Stanek, 2019). In contrast, the main drawback of laser angioplasty is that current laser catheters cannot create a sufficiently wide channel in the blood vessel, meaning that supplementary balloon dilatation is still required (Stanek, 2019). For the application of lasers in the field of laser angioplasty, it is essential to consider not only the laser itself but also the whole laser system. This system consists of a laser, a connector, a laser catheter, and a catheter tip. The connector acts as a guide to direct the laser light into the laser catheter. The laser catheter is composed of one or more optical fibres, which transmit the laser energy. The catheter tip is an essential component of the laser system and may be crucial for the success of the laser procedure (Stanek, 2019). Laser angioplasty is a safe method, as the complication rate does not exceed that of standard angioplasty. However, it does have a higher cost which is an obvious barrier to accessibility (Stanek, 2019).

The excimer laser was launched in clinical practice in the 1990s when optical fibres for the transmission of radiation from the excimer laser became available (Stanek, 2019). Its name originates from a combination of "excited" and "dimer." Excimer lasers ("excimers") are a potent source of UV energy, which are very well absorbed by tissue proteins and lipids. The mechanism of action of excimers is nonthermal ("cool lasers"). Thus, they cause precise ablation of tissues without thermal damage (Stanek, 2019). However, the use of the excimer laser in patients with the peripheral arterial disease was only approved for use by the Food and Drug Administration in the USA in 2003 (Stanek, 2019).

One severe but rare complication of angioplasty is iatrogenic coronary artery perforation (CAP) due to underlying complex lesions. Iatrogenic coronary artery perforation is rare and hazardous, almost always resulting in death, occurring in only 0.1% to 0.8 % of cases (Chhabra, 2020). In addition, in-stent restenosis is defined as reducing vascular luminal diameter after the procedure done through the skin. The underlying physiological processes associated with in-stent restenosis depend on the type of stent used during angioplasty. A meta-analysis showed that patients with unstable angina or acute coronary syndrome who underwent an angioplasty were more likely to develop in-stent restenosis due to chronic inflammation, which was predicted by a higher C-reactive protein level (CRP). Therefore, a C-creative protein test is done to detect inflammation in these patients compared to patients with stable angina (Chhabra, 2020). Lastly, specific risk factors are associated with age, acuity of presentation and the baseline of other comorbidities such as diabetes or chronic lung disease (Watson et al., 2018).

To sum, angioplasty is a non-invasive procedure used to target blood vessels infected with plaque. Furthermore, due to the reality that heart disease and strokes are a leading cause of mortality and morbidity in developed countries worldwide. Ongoing treatment of atherosclerosis with stents and lasers has contributed to an overall increase in quality of life for those tormented with blood vessels bound for obstruction. As a result, healthcare providers are able to eliminate the obstructions to the vessels relieving the patient and allowing the blood to transport oxygen to the body. Therefore, understanding angioplasty resides in understanding the critical mechanical elements and their role in treating ventricle obstructions.

RECENT SIGNIFICANCE IN MEDICINE

As human longevity continues to increase, two of the most common causes of death in Canada have become cardiovascular diseases and cancer. As these two health problems cause many deaths in Canada every year, it is essential that treatments that work and offer patients a high quality of life are developed and refined for these two conditions. Concerning cardiovascular disease, one treatment that is frequently used is angioplasty. This procedure is used in several different scenarios and has helped save the lives of many patients and increase their longevity and quality of life. Staying informed about treatments for cardiovascular disease is essential both for current health care providers, future health care providers and the general population as it is likely that everyone will know someone who will suffer from a form of cardiovascular disease at some point in their lifetime.

Angioplasty is a surgical procedure that can open blocked coronary arteries (Hopkins, n.d.). The purpose of angioplasty is to open the blocked coronary arteries so that blood flow to the heart will be restored without open-heart surgery (Hopkins, n.d.). If blood flow is not fixed to the heart, there is a risk of the cardiac muscle not receiving enough nutrients and oxygen, which can cause it to die (Hopkins, n.d.). This would be a myocardial infarct, otherwise known as a heart attack. One of the significant benefits of angioplasty is that it is much less risky than open-heart surgery, as the thoracic cavity does not need to be opened (Hopkins, n.d.). Instead, a long thin tube, known as a catheter, will be put into a blood vessel (Hopkins, n.d.). This catheter is unique because it has a tiny balloon at its tip (Hopkins, n.d.). The catheter will then be guided through the blood vessels to the blocked coronary artery. Once the catheter has reached the narrowed area of the blocked coronary artery, the balloon will be inflated (Hopkins, n.d.). This will exert pressure on the obstruction (often plaque or a blood clot) and push the plaque/blood clot against the sides of the artery, which allows for more room in the artery for blood to flow through (Hopkins, n.d.). This can help ensure a steady blood flow through the coronary artery, ensuring that the heart's cardiac muscle is getting enough nutrients and oxygen and ensuring that waste products are removed (Hopkins, n.d.).

Fluoroscopy is used to guide the catheter through the blood vessels. Fluoroscopy is a type of X-ray technology in which a continuous X-ray is passed through the body part being examined (Hopkins, n.d.). In the case of angioplasty, the fluoroscopy would be imaging the blood vessels. Before the procedure, a contrast dye will move through the arteries, allowing the arteries to be easily visualized (Hopkins, n.d.). The beam will then be transmitted to a monitor, which will let the healthcare provider operating the angioplasty see the blood vessel the catheter is passing through (Hopkins, n.d.). Since it is a continuous X-ray beam, the healthcare provider will see the catheter as it moves through the blood vessels, which is ideal to ensure that the health care provider can control the catheter (Hopkins, n.d.).

That is the basic procedure for balloon angioplasty, but there are also other types of angioplasties. For example, another similar angioplasty procedure is called an atherectomy, which involves removing the plaque from the narrowed coronary artery (Hopkins, n.d.). This procedure follows a very similar premise to balloon angioplasty. Still, instead of a catheter with a tiny balloon at the end, a catheter with a rotating tip will be inserted into the artery (Hopkins, n.d.). When the catheter reaches the narrowed spot, the rotating end will break up the plaque to open up the artery, which increases blood flow through the artery (Hopkins, n.d.).

Now that the artery has been reopened, it is essential to ensure that it will not narrow or close again. To do this, coronary stents are used (Hopkins, n.d.). A stent can be thought of as a very small, expandable, metal mesh coil (Hopkins, n.d.). Once the artery has been reopened, a stent will often be placed at the site of the balloon angioplasty to ensure that the artery does not narrow or close again (Hopkins, n.d.). Since the stent is a foreign object to the body, once it has been inserted in the body, the body will begin to coat the stent with tissue (Hopkins, n.d.). Within three months to one year, the stent will be fully lined with tissue (Hopkins, n.d.). However, this can be problematic if scar tissue forms inside the stent, so most stents are now coated with medicine to prevent this (Hopkins, n.d.).

These medicine-coated stents are called drug-eluting stents (DES), and they slow the overgrowth of tissue within the stent by releasing the drug into the blood vessel (Hopkins, n.d.). While it is good that these stents minimize the rates of stenosis and prevent the blood vessel from narrowing again, they can increase the presence of platelets in the blood vessel (Hopkins, n.d.). Since the function of platelets is to form blood clots to stop bleeding, having more platelets present can increase the likelihood of a blood clot in the coronary artery (Hopkins, n.d.). A blood clot in a coronary artery could cause a heart attack, which would be very dangerous to the patient. To reduce the risk of a heart attack occurring, patients with drug-eluting stents are often prescribed antiplatelet medicines that need to be taken for an extended time (Hopkins, n.d.). Since this can be dangerous for people who have a high risk of bleeding (antiplatelets reduce blood clotting, so they increase the risk of uncontrolled bleeding), some people get stents that are not coated in medicine (Hopkins, n.d.). These stents are called bare-metal stents (BMS) (Hopkins, n.d.). These stents have a higher risk of stenosis because more scar tissue forms inside the stent, but patients with bare-metal stents will not require long-term use of antiplatelets, which will reduce their risk of uncontrolled internal bleeding (Hopkins, n.d.). However, if too much scar tissue forms inside the stent, the coronary artery will be blocked again, meaning another procedure will be needed (Hopkins, n.d.). This often means undergoing a second balloon angioplasty with a second stent to open up the artery again (Hopkins, n.d.). Another angioplasty option would be to use radiation therapy, which is called brachytherapy (Hopkins, n.d.). This would be done through a catheter placed close to the scar tissue (Hopkins, n.d.). The radiation therapy should stop the growth of the scar tissue and open up the coronary artery (Hopkins, n.d.).

Now that the basic principles of angioplasty are understood, in what scenarios would angioplasty be needed. When can angioplasty be used? There are several answers to this question as angioplasty can be used in a variety of situations. One of the most common situations in which angioplasty is used has already been mentioned above: to open up a coronary vessel that has accumulated a buildup of fatty plaques (Levine et al., 2016). The disease where there is a buildup of fatty plaques in blood vessels is called atherosclerosis (Levine et al., 2016). Angioplasty is usually only recommended to patients who have already tried medications or lifestyle changes but have not seen any improvements in their condition because it is a more invasive treatment and is therefore much riskier (Levine et al., 2016). Alternatively, angioplasty can also be used in emergencies, such as if worsening angina (chest pain) is present or if the patient is having a heart attack (Levine et al., 2016). Angioplasty is helpful for patients who are having a heart attack because it can quickly and effectively open the blocked artery (Levine et al., 2016). This allows blood to flow to one's heart, provides the heart with nutrients and oxygen, and removes waste products from the heart (Levine et al., 2016). This will reduce the total damage to one's heart. If a heart attack has already happened, opening up the blocked artery as quickly as possible is vital to ensure that the heart does not suffer too much damage to function (Levine et al., 2016).

However, angioplasty is a somewhat invasive procedure and therefore does have some risks. The three most common risks of angioplasty are having the artery re-narrow, having a blood clot at the angioplasty site, and bleeding (Levine et al., 2016). The risk of having the artery re-narrow can be mitigated by using a drug-eluting stent, as discussed above. The risk of blood clots can be minimized by prescribing the patient antiplatelet therapy (Levine et al., 2016). In addition, bleeding can occur in the area where the catheter was inserted, which would usually be an arm or a leg (Levine et al., 2016). A bleeding complication is usually not too severe. It often only results in a bruise at the insertion site, but occasionally more severe bleeding can occur, so that surgical procedures or even a blood transfusion may be required (Levine et al., 2016). There are also several rarer risks from an angioplasty, such as having a heart attack during the procedure, having a coronary artery be torn or ruptured by the procedure, or having a stroke. A stroke can occur because some of the plaques on the blood vessel walls can break loose when the catheter is threaded through the aorta (Levine et al., 2016). These plaques can then travel to the brain and block blood flow there, which causes a stroke (Levine et al., 2016). In addition, abnormal heart rhythms during the procedure, such as the heart beating either too quickly or too slowly, can also occur, but this problem is usually not long-term (Levine et al., 2016). However, a temporary pacemaker or medications might sometimes be needed to mitigate the irregular heart rhythms (Levine et al., 2016). Finally, kidney problems can also occur because of the contrast dye used during the angioplasty (Levine et al., 2016).

There are still many complications that can occur during angioplasty. For this reason, it is essential to continue to innovate and try to find ways to make angioplasty safer and more effective. In recent years, there have been several new advancements related to coronary angioplasty. One aspect of the procedure that has improved is the intravascular imaging techniques (Cardiologist, 2019). One such technique is optical coherence tomography (Cardiologist, 2019). Optical coherence tomography gives the healthcare provider more information on the plaque that blocks the vessel, such as if it is hard or soft and consists of lipids or calcium (Cardiologist, 2019). This can help decide the size of the stent needed and help when health care providers are checking the vessel's status after the stent has been placed (Cardiologist, 2019). Optical coherence tomography works by using light near the infrared spectrum to create images of the inside of the coronary arteries (Texas Heart Institute, n.d.). The advantage to using this technique is that visuals with a high resolution are produced (Texas Heart Institute, n.d.). These high-resolution images are produced because optical coherence tomography reduces the amount of glare from scattered light (Texas Heart Institute, n.d.). This means that all the reflected light can be detected and used to form a high-resolution image of the desired coronary artery (Texas Heart Institute, n.d.). This works to the extent that using optical coherence tomography produces an image ten times more detailed than an intravascular ultrasound (Texas Heart Institute, n.d.).

Another new technique that has helped make angioplasties safer is fractional flow reserve (FRR), a tool that can assess if angioplasty is needed (Cardiologist, 2019). It can help healthcare providers decide if an angioplasty and stent would be ideal or if the patient would be better suited to another treatment method such as bypass surgery or a medication-based treatment (Cardiologist, 2019). Fractional flow reserve is a ratio that compares the maximum flow of blood through the coronary artery that is blocked to the standard full flow in that coronary artery without blockage or stenosis (Pijls et al., 1995). These values are calculated by measuring the mean arterial, distal coronary and ventral venous pressure at the same time while also inducing vasodilation pharmacologically (using drugs to cause the arteries and veins to dilate) (Pijls et al., 1995). Once the ratio is obtained, the health care provider can determine the severity of the stenosis, which can help the healthcare provider choose the right treatment plan (Pijls et al., 1995).

Another new angioplasty technique uses a bioresorbable vascular scaffold (BVS) instead of a stent (Cardiologist, 2019). The bioresorbable vascular scaffold functions similarly to a stent except for the fact that it can dissolve when the previously blocked artery no longer needs the stents to stay open (Cardiologist, 2019). This can reduce scar tissue buildup and decrease the need for a second angioplasty (Cardiologist, 2019). The goal of using the bioresorbable vascular scaffold was to have a stent that would not disrupt further treatments and allow normal coronary vasomotion after the procedure has been completed (Jinnouchi, 2019). In addition, it should also decrease long-term foreign body response (Jinnouchi, 2019). Unfortunately, the results from clinical trials using these stents have not been promising, as a patient who had received the bioresorbable vascular scaffold had had higher rates of myocardial infarction due to a blockage in the artery with the bioresorbable vascular scaffold, as well as higher rates of stent thrombosis (a blood clot in the stent) compared to the metallic drug-eluting stents that were used before the bioresorbable vascular scaffold was introduced (Jinnouchi, 2019). Due to these complications, it would appear that the bioresorbable vascular scaffold still needs some modifications before it can have the desired results. However, it is still an innovative treatment option, even if it is not ideal (Jinnouchi, 2019).

While it is impressive that all these new developments and innovations have occurred in the field of angioplasty, the original technique of using a balloon catheter remains popular to this day. Luckily, there have been several recent advances to balloon catheters that have allowed them to become more effective and reduce complications (DAIC, 2021). One such example is the introduction of drug-coated balloons, otherwise known as drug-eluting balloons (DAIC, 2021). Drug-coated balloons function similarly to drug-eluting stents, as they contain the same drugs (DAIC, 2021). The advantage to drug-coated balloons is that they can prevent the vessel from re-occluding due to the buildup of scar tissue, which can otherwise occur due to the angioplasty balloons tearing and stretching the vessel lining when they expand (DAIC, 2021). Some other advancements to this device are that some balloons now have nitinol wire wrapped around the balloon (DAIC, 2021). The purpose of this is to increase the pressure to cut calcified lesions (DAIC, 2021). Doing this will help the stent to expand fully (DAIC, 2021). This type of treatment usually is only used when the original balloon does not break the calcium enough to expand properly (DAIC, 2021). Finally, recently, the shockwave intravascular lithotripsy system has been introduced (DAIC, 2021). This system includes a regular balloon on the catheter, with the catheter delivering bursts of sonic energy to crack the calcium (DAIC, 2021). The sonic energy can be thought of like sound waves powerful enough to shatter the calcium that is occluding the vessel (DAIC, 2021).

Overall, angioplasty has been a revolutionary discovery that has changed how healthcare providers and cardiologists treat occluded coronary arteries, heart disease and heart attacks. While the angioplasty balloon had remained one of the favoured treatments since it was introduced when angioplasty was developed, there have since been numerous advancements in the technology that allow increased visualization of the coronary arteries, that minimize the complications caused by the procedure and that increase the effectiveness of the angioplasty balloon. Some examples of these improvements were discussed in this chapter, such as the drug-eluting stents, drug-coated balloons and optical coherence tomography. Furthermore, some of these advancements are good starting points but still need some work to be perfected, such as the bioresorbable vascular scaffold. While complications still exist and the procedure could be improved, the advancements made on angioplasty since it has been introduced to the medical field have helped improve and save many lives. In addition, they have made a difference for those suffering from and who will suffer from various cardiovascular diseases. It is exciting to see what the future will bring for this exciting field!

CHAPTER 6 | KARANVEER KAUSHAL
ANGIOPLASTY OPERATIONS AND THE SCIENCE BEHIND IT

Angioplasty, also known as balloon angioplasty or percutaneous translumi-nal angioplasty (PTA), is a minimally invasive endovascular procedure for widening narrowed or obstructed arteries or veins (Waqas, 2019). It's most commonly used to treat arterial atherosclerosis (sometimes called "hardening" or "clogging" of the arteries). A balloon catheter (a deflated balloon attached to a catheter) is passed into the narrowed vessel over a guidewire and then inflated to the appropriate size of the clogged artery. The balloon causes the blood vessel and the surrounding muscular wall to expand, allowing for better blood flow. A stent may be inserted during ballooning to keep the artery intact structurally, and so the arty won't be clogged again, after which the balloon is deflated and removed (Waqas, 2019). Angioplasty has come to include all vascular interventions typically performed percutaneously (Waqas, 2019).

A coronary angiogram and X-ray with radio-opaque contrast in the cor-onary arteries shows the left coronary circulation. The distal left main coronary artery (LMCA) is in the left upper quadrant of the image (Cilin-giroglu, 2019). Its main branches also visible are the left circumflex artery (LCX), which courses top-to-bottom initially and then toward the centre bottom, and the left anterior descending (LAD) artery, which courses from left-to-right on the image and then courses down the middle of the image to project underneath the distal LCX. The LAD, as is usual, has two large diagonal branches, which arise at the centre-top of the image and course toward the centre-right of the picture (Cilingiroglu, 2019).

A coronary angioplasty is a therapeutic procedure to treat the stenotic (narrowed) coronary arteries of the heart found in coronary heart disease (Cilingiroglu, 2019). These stenotic segments of the coronary arteries arise due to the buildup of cholesterol-laden plaques that form in a condition known as atherosclerosis (Cilingiroglu, 2019). A percutaneous coronary intervention (PCI), or coronary angioplasty with stenting, is a non-surgical procedure used to improve the blood flow to the heart (Cilingiroglu, 2019).

Coronary Angioplasty is indicated for coronary artery diseases such as unstable angina, NSTEMI, STEMI and spontaneous coronary artery perforation. PCI for the stable coronary disease has been shown to significantly relieve symptoms such as angina, or chest pain, thereby improving functional limitations and quality of life (Cilingiroglu, 2019).

CHRONIC LIMB-THREATENING ISCHEMIA

Angioplasty is a procedure that may be used to treat progressive peripheral artery disease and alleviate the claudication, or leg pain, that is often associated with the condition (Balk, 2016).

In the bypass versus angioplasty in profound ischemia of the leg (BASIL) study, select patients with severe lower limb ischemia who were eligible for either operation were compared to bypass surgery first versus angioplasty. The BASIL trial discovered that angioplasty was associated with less short-term morbidity than bypass surgery but had better long-term results (Balk, 2016).

RENAL ARTERY ANGIOPLASTY

The ACCF/AHA recommendations prescribe balloon angioplasty only for patients with a life expectancy of fewer than two years or who do not have an autogenous vein available, based on the findings of the BASIL study (Gregory, 2013). A bypass surgery could be done first on patients with a life expectancy of more than two years or who have an autogenous vein (Gregory, 2013).

CAROTID ANGIOPLASTY

For patients at high risk of carotid endarterectomy, carotid artery stenosis should be treated with angioplasty and carotid stenting (CEA) (Chong, 2019). Although carotid endarterectomy is usually favoured to carotid artery stenting, stenting may be necessary for certain patients with radiation-induced stenosis or a carotid lesion that is not amenable to surgery (Chong, 2019).

VENOUS ANGIOPLASTY

Angioplasty is used to treat venous stenosis that affects hemodialysis entry, with drug-coated balloon angioplasty proving to be more effective than traditional balloon angioplasty at 6 and 12 months (Chong, 2019). Following thoracic outlet decompression surgery for thoracic outlet syndrome, angioplasty is occasionally used to treat latent subclavian vein stenosis. In addition, there is a weak recommendation for deep venous stenting to treat obstructive chronic venous disease (Chong, 2019).

CONTRAINDICATIONS

An access vessel, usually the femoral or radial artery or the femoral vein, is required for angioplasty to allow wires and catheters access to the vascular system (Chong, 2019). Angioplasty is not recommended where there is no suitable access vessel of appropriate size and consistency. For example, a small vessel diameter, the presence of posterior calcification, occlusion, hematoma, or an earlier placement of a bypass origin, may make access to the vascular system too tricky (Chong, 2019). In addition, percutaneous transluminal coronary angioplasty (PTCA) is contraindicated in patients with left primary coronary artery disease due to the risk of spasm of the left main coronary artery during the procedure. Also, PTCA is not recommended if there is less than 70% stenosis of the coronary arteries, as the stenosis is not deemed to be hemodynamically significant below this level (Chong, 2019).

Angioplasty without stenting was related to a considerable danger of restenosis, which prompted interest in angioplasty with stenting. Inflatable mounted coronary stents, notwithstanding, are restricted by the high expansion pressures required for the organization in delicate intracranial vessels and the danger of shearing the stent from the inflatable while exploring to the objective sore (DAIC, 2021). These stents were related with generally high paces of specialized disappointment because of the convolution of the intracranial dissemination and the overall solidness of coronary stages; for fruitful methods, the paces of periprocedural dreariness and mortality were acceptable.20-22 Jiang et al.22 announced a specialized achievement rate (characterized as equivalent to 20% leftover stenosis) of 97.6%, with a 10% significant complexity rate in 40 patients with 42 suggestive M1 stenotic injuries treated with angioplasty and inflatable mounted coronary stents (DAIC, 2021).

ANGIOPLASTY OF THE CEREBRAL VASCULATURE

Angioplasty alludes to a strategy of extending a limited course by expanding an inflatable inside the limited area. This method is generally performed by the percutaneous inclusion of an inflatable catheter through a removed vessel (generally the femoral conduit). As needs are, it is known as percutaneous transluminal angioplasty (PTA). Angioplasty might be performed for blood vessel narrowing from various causes, including the fit of the veins (vasospasm) and "solidifying of the supply routes" (atherosclerosis). The most well-known destinations for treating atherosclerotic narrowing in the cerebrovascular framework are the vertebral and carotid conduits in the neck (Kokkinidis, 2018). Angioplasty for atherosclerotic narrowing of the carotid supply routes is quickly getting acknowledged as an effective treatment to forestall stroke. Two enormous, randomized multicenter preliminaries have demonstrated that careful fix of an extraordinarily limited (i.e., 70% or more) carotid supply route (endarterectomy) diminishes the danger stroke in chosen patients. In any case, this advantage may not be inferred by patients considered a danger for a medical procedure or general sedation because the dangers for perioperative difficulties are additionally huge. With expanding recurrence, such "high-hazard" patients are currently considered for angioplasty of unhealthy courses. Likewise, patients with massive narrowing at the beginning of the vertebral vein may profit from endovascular treatment because careful fixation can be more dangerous in the vertebral Artery than in the carotid supply route. Angioplasty improves the patency of a vein limited by atherosclerotic plaque by breaking the plaque and extending the media of the vessel divider. Consequently, the vessel divider is rebuilt by regrowth of the inward coating, or intima, which covers the broken plaque. At most establishments, angioplasty is combined with the arrangement of a stent. The stent may diminish the danger of deferred restenosis at the angioplasty site and lessen the danger of injury to the conduit during angioplasty. Subsequently, numerous endovascular specialists utilize inflatable angioplasty to open the vein enough to put the stent and perform complete widening once the stent is set up (Kokkinidis, 2018).

The significant danger of carotid or vertebral conduit angioplasty is stroke, which happens during or after angioplasty in around 1–5% of patients. Stroke may result from bits of the plaque that sever and embolize intracranial vessels and block the bloodstream. For example, distal security is expanding an inflatable distal to the treatment site to obstruct the stream briefly and thus wash emboli from the interior carotid conduit to the outside carotid vein of the face, which may lessen this danger. New distal security gadgets being scrutinized utilize a channel that catches emboli without blocking the bloodstream. Stroke may likewise result from blood clusters that structure on the recently broken plaque or metal stent. The utilization of medications to restrain cluster arrangement, particularly antiplatelet specialists, has limited thickening entanglements. Early reports demonstrate that wellbeing and viability are like those of endarterectomy, especially for high-hazard careful patients. A vast, imminent preliminary is in progress to analyze the two strategies (Messina, 2004).

Angioplasty in the intracranial course may likewise be considered for the treatment of atherosclerosis. Albeit no enormous preliminaries have been performed to help anticipate which patients will infer the best advantage, those with transient indications identified with a limited conduit are generally viewed as the best applicants (Dueck, 2019). The presence of side effects in a patient without a vast, finished infarct shows that the patient is in danger for future occasions, including stroke (Dueck, 2019). At the same time, cerebrum tissue and, in this way, capacity might be salvageable. Similar standards of angioplasty in the extracranial course apply to the intracranial dissemination (Dueck, 2019). As it may, the more modest size of the objective vessels intracranially puts impediments on the endovascular procedure. Troubles or threats related to propelling a stent through a limited intracranial vessel regularly require treatment by expanding angioplasty alone. What's more, distal branches might be tiny in any event for angioplasty. At present, branches distal to the carotid bifurcation or proximal center cerebral supply route in the front flow. The basilar or proximal back cerebral courses in the back dissemination are viewed as an exceptional danger. They are once in a while treated with angioplasty. Another site often treated with angioplasty and stenting is the subclavian conduit. Stenosis of the subclavian line may bring about a wonder known as subclavian take. In the present circumstance, the bloodstream to the arm is limited to such an extent that the stream in the vertebral vein might be turned around, streaming lower and out to the arm. Subclavian conditions may cause vertebrobasilar deficiency, with dizziness, visual side effects, loss of awareness, or any mix of these. Fixing the stenosis regularly turns around the "take." It improves the patient's indications (Dueck, 2019).

Angioplasty is a minimally invasive surgical procedure used to open block blood vessels that travel to the heart. Also called a percutaneous transluminal coronary angioplasty (PTCA) or percutaneous coronary intervention (PCI), the procedure is often performed after an episode of chest pain or a heart attack and typically involves the placement of a stent(Widimsky, 2010). Angioplasty may not be suitable for everyone. Patients with several blockages in certain places, or total occlusion of the artery may need coronary bypass instead. The procedure is also contraindicated for people with particular bleeding and coagulation disorders and those who may be allergic to contrast dye (Widimsky, 2010).

Doctors can diagnose atherosclerosis and CAD using imaging tests, such as echocardiography, computed tomography (CT) scan, magnetic resonance imaging (MRI), positron emission tomography (PET), or angiography (Oldroyd, 2017). Mild cases are typically treated with statins and heart-healthy lifestyle changes to lower cholesterol. More severe cases of atherosclerosis require surgery, and angioplasty is the most common procedure used to treat clogged arteries and improve blood flow to the heart. It is one of the most common procedures performed in the United States each year. Angioplasty does not correct atherosclerosis; it only relieves related blockages(Oldroyd, 2017). However, angioplasty is quite effective in reducing the symptoms of stable angina and is often used in treating coronary artery disease in people who have acute coronary syndrome (ACS). In ACS, acute blockage of a coronary artery occurs due to a ruptured plaque that has formed a clot within the artery. When this happens, a heart attack is very likely unless the artery is opened. Angioplasty and stenting can help during such an event to improve overall cardiac outcomes. Other surgical options for treating atherosclerosis include coronary artery bypass grafting (CABG) and carotid endarterectomy (Oldroyd, 2017).

Before one will have an angioplasty, the doctor will perform a complete medical history and physical exam, likely this procedure will require a chest X-ray, electrocardiogram, and blood tests prior to the patient going into the surgery itself (Oldroyd, 2017). In assessing the appropriate course of treatment for one's condition, the cardiologist may perform an angiogram—a procedure that uses contrast dye and X-ray to visualize arterial blockages (Oldroyd, 2017). This test is used in determining if one or more stents may be required. If angioplasty is performed as an urgent procedure during an acute or impending heart attack, an angiogram will be done in conjunction with the angioplasty as a single procedure (Oldroyd, 2017). Refer to a doctor about the potential risks and benefits for the patient personally and other potential treatment options.

Angioplasty is performed while the patient is awake. The procedure is not painful, and no incision will be made. The procedure can take anywhere from 30 minutes to three hours, depending on the number of blockages that need to be treated and any complications that may arise. Once the anesthesia has taken effect, the surgical staff will sterilize the skin where the catheter will be inserted—the brachial artery in the arm, the radial artery in the wrist, or the femoral artery in the groin. The area will also likely be covered with a cellophane-like sheet. After numbing the area, the doctor will insert a needle into the artery. Using the exact opening, they will then insert a catheter. Live X-rays help guide the surgeon to the heart, where a contrast dye will be injected to highlight the blockages (Tarantini et al., 2010). Next, the doctor will insert another catheter with a deflated balloon and, if needed, a stent to open a blocked artery. Once the catheter reaches the blockage, the balloon is inflated to compress the plaque against the artery wall (Tarantini et al., 2010). The balloon is then deflated, and any stents are placed. The doctor will determine the type of stent to use: either a bare-metal stent or a drug-eluting stent, a metal mesh coated with a slow-releasing medicine to prevent the artery from narrowing again. Different types of drug-eluting stents are coated with different medicines. After the angioplasty is finished, the surgeon will quickly remove the catheter and use a particular device to close the artery (Tarantini et al., 2010).

CORONARY ANGIOPLASTY PROCEDURES: WHAT RESEARCHERS DON'T KNOW

Angioplasty is a procedure for removing fatty plaques from the blood vessels of the heart (Tarantini et al., 2010). Atherosclerosis is a form of heart disease characterized by an accumulation of plaque. If one has taken medications and made lifestyle changes yet it has not improved cardiovascular health, angioplasty is a good option for treating the disease (Tarantini et al., 2010). For example, if one is experiencing increased chest pain (angina), it may have been a heart attack. Angioplasty can open a blocked artery rapidly, minimizing heart damage; however, not everybody is a candidate for angioplasty. One doctor can decide that coronary artery bypass surgery is a better choice than angioplasty, depending on the severity of the individual's heart disease and one's overall health (Tarantini et al., 2010). For example, suppose the main artery supplying blood to the left side of the heart is narrowed. In that case, coronary artery bypass surgery may be necessary if one has weak heart muscle, diabetes, and severe artery blockages (Tarantini et al., 2010). A safe blood vessel from another part of the body is used to bypass the blocked portion of the artery during coronary artery bypass surgery (Tarantini et al., 2010).

A balloon is used to open a clogged coronary (heart) artery narrowed due to atherosclerosis. This treatment improves the supply of blood to the heart. Plaque builds up on the inner walls of the arteries, causing atherosclerosis. Any artery, including the coronary arteries, which carry oxygen-rich blood to the heart, may be affected. Coronary artery disease is the result of atherosclerosis affecting the coronary arteries (CAD) (Tarantini et al., 2010). Angioplasty can be used for various purposes, including Reduce CAD symptoms, including angina and shortness of breath (Tarantini et al., 2010). If a coronary artery is completely blocked, a heart attack occurs, and after a heart attack, angioplasty can lessen the damage to the heart muscle. As a result, some patients' chances of dying are reduced. In the United States, angioplasties are performed on over a million people every year. Serious complications are uncommon, but they can occur regardless of how cautious the doctor is or how well the procedure is performed (Tarantini et al., 2010). Angioplasty research is underway to make the operation safer and more efficient and prevent treated arteries from closing again and make the procedure more accessible to a broader range of people (Tarantini et al., 2010).

While angioplasty is a less invasive procedure than bypass surgery, it still has some risks. Angioplasty has several threats; the most critical threat that doctors are constantly trying to avoid is the artery reblocking again (Tarantini et al., 2010). Although the treated artery has a slight chance of being blocked again by the addition of a stent, it has an even higher chance of blocking with an insertion of a drug-eluting stent; however, the possibility of this happening is less than 5% (Tarantini et al., 2010). The formation of blood clots is also prevalent in angioplasty, which can potentially block an artery and cause problems such as heart attack or stroke (Tarantini et al., 2010). To minimize the risk of clots forming in a stent, doctors recommend aspirin in conjunction with clopidogrel (Plavix), prasugrel (Effient), or other drugs that help prevent blood clots (Tarantini et al., 2010). The variety and dosage of each drug correspond with the individual being treated, so one needs to consult with a medical professional for a prescription (Tarantini et al., 2010). Finally, an individual may experience bleeding where the catheter was implanted in one's leg or arm. Usually, this only causes a bruise, but severe bleeding can occur, necessitating a blood transfusion or surgical procedures (Tarantini et al., 2010).

Heart attack is a rare side effect of angioplasty. There is a rare chance that one may suffer from a heart attack during the operation; however, this is a rare occurrence and is extremely unlikely (Tarantini et al., 2010). Coronary artery disease is a condition that occurs when the arteries in the heart. During the procedure, the coronary artery may be ripped or ruptured. These complications could necessitate bypass surgery as soon as possible. In addition, there could be potential Kidney issues. The dye used during angioplasty and stent placement can harm the kidneys, particularly in people with kidney issues (Tarantini et al., 2010). If one is at a higher risk, a medical professional can take precautions to protect the kidneys, such as reducing the amount of contrast dye used and ensuring that the patient is well-hydrated during the procedure (Tarantini et al., 2010).

Stroke is a medical term that describes a condition in which plaque blocks blood flow to the heart; when the catheters are threaded through the aorta during angioplasty, plaques may break free and reduce blood flow and cause strokes (Widimsky, 2010). Blood clots can occur in catheters as well, and if they break free, they can migrate to the brain (Widimsky, 2010). Since a stroke is a rare complication of coronary angioplasty, blood thinners reduce the likelihood of irregular heart rhythms during the procedure. As a result, the heart can beat too quickly or too slowly during the procedure (Widimsky, 2010). These heart rhythm issues are rare and generally temporary, but medications or a temporary pacemaker may be required to fix the problem (Widimsky, 2010).

Angioplasty is performed by a heart-trained professional (cardiologist) and a group of specific cardiovascular medical caretakers and experts in an exceptional working room called a cardiovascular catheterization research facility (Wilson et al., 2017). Angioplasty is performed through one's crotch, arm or wrist territory. An exciting thing about Angioplasty is that general sedation isn't required; patients will be given a narcotic to help them relax; however, they will most likely remain conscious throughout the procedure (Wilson et al., 2017). Medical professionals will also administer liquids and drugs such as anticoagulants through an IV in one arm. The patient's pulse rate, circulatory strain and oxygen levels will all be observed during the surgery (Wilson et al., 2017). The primary care physician will set up space in the patient's leg, arm or wrist with a disinfectant arrangement and put a sterile sheet over one's body. Next, the primary care physician will utilize a sedative to numb the region where a small cut will be made. A tiny slim guidewire is then embedded in the vein. With the assistance of live X- beams, the primary care physician will string a cylinder (catheter) through one's circulatory system (Wilson et al., 2017). The different colour is infused through the catheter once it is set up, which permits the doctor to see within the veins and recognize the blockage on X-beam pictures called angiograms. A little inflatable with or without a stent at the tip of the catheter is swelled at the sight of the blockage, broadening the hindered artery. After the artery is expanded, the inflatable balloon is flattened, and the catheter is taken out (Wilson et al., 2017). If one has a few blockages, the technique might be rehashed at every stoppage (Wilson et al., 2017). Angioplasty can take as long as a few hours, contingent upon the trouble and number of jams and whether any entanglements emerge (Wilson et al., 2017).

WHAT OCCURS AFTER ANGIOPLASTY?

In the medical clinic after the procedure, one might be taken to the recuperation space for perception or go back to the medical clinic room. The patient will remain level in bed for a few hours after the methodology (Liebetrau et al., 2017). A medical caretaker will screen the patient for crucial signs, the additional site, and dissemination and sensation in the influenced leg or arm. If the patient feels any chest agony or snugness, or some other torment, a medical professional should be let known as they are the best fit to deal with situations. Bed rest may differ from 2 to 6 hours relying upon the patient's particular condition (Liebetrau et al., 2017). Patients' bed rest can be restricted if their primary care physician prescribes a conclusion device. The medical attendant will help the patient on the first occasion when they get up and check their circulatory strain while lying in bed, sitting, and standing (Liebetrau et al., 2017). The patient is advised to move gradually while getting up to stay away from any dizziness from the extensive stretch of bed rest (Liebetrau et al., 2017). The patient might be given torment medication for agony or distress at the addition site or lying level and still for quite a while (Liebetrau et al., 2017).

The patient will be urged to drink water and different liquids to help flush the different colours from the body. In the end, they may return their standard eating routine after the system unless the primary care physician chooses something else (Liebetrau et al., 2017). The patient will undoubtedly go through the night in the clinic after the procedure. Contingent upon their condition and the after-effects of the procedure, the patient's visit might be longer. Once at home, a small wound is ordinary; however, on the off chance that one notices a steady measure of blood at the site, it can be contained with a dressing; however, it would be wise to let a medical practitioner know (Liebetrau et al., 2017).

If a primary care physician utilized a conclusion gadget at the patient's inclusion site, the patient would be provided detailed data concerning a sense of finality gadget that was utilized and how to deal with the site (Wilson et al., 2017). There will be a little bunch, or irregularity, under the skin at the site (Wilson et al., 2017). This is typical. The bunch ought to gradually vanish over half a month. It will be imperative to keep the inclusion site spotless and dry (Wilson et al., 2017). The medical services group will give the patient explicit washing directions. It would be wise to let the skin around the wound heal before submerging it into pools of water (Wilson et al., 2017). It would also be advised to not partake in any strenuous exercises until further notice (Wilson et al., 2017).

THE PATIENT SHOULD TELL THE DOCTOR IF THEY HAVE ANY OF THE ACCOMPANYING:

Fever or chills, Expanded torment, redness, growing, dying, or other waste from the addition site, Coolness, deadness or shivering, or different changes in the influenced arm or leg (Liebetrau et al., 2017). Chest agony or critical factors like queasiness or heaving, abundant perspiring, wooziness, or blacking out should also be told to doctors (Liebetrau et al., 2017).

BEFORE A PATIENT CONSENTS TO THE TEST OR THE TECHNIQUE, ALL PATIENTS MUST KNOW:

The name of the test or technique, The explanation of having the test or technique, what are the results to expectations and what they mean, the dangers and advantages of the test or technique, what the possible results or entanglements are, when and where the patient will have the test or technique, who will do the test or technique and what that individual's capabilities are, what might occur on the off chance that one doesn't get the test or methodology, any elective tests or techniques to consider, how the outcomes will be, who to call after the test or technique if the patient has questions or issues and lastly, the amount one should pay for the test or methodology (Liebetrau et al., 2017). The discoveries of an enormous government concentrate on sidestep medical procedures and stents raise doubt about the clinical consideration given to a vast number of coronary illness patients with impeded coronary courses, researchers detailed at the yearly gathering of the American Heart Association on Saturday (Liebetrau et al., 2017).

The new examination found that patients who got drug treatment alone didn't encounter more respiratory failures or pass on more regularly than the individuals who additionally got sidestep a medical procedure or stents, minuscule wire confines used to open narrow arteries (Liebetrau et al., 2017). That discovery remained constant for patients with a few seriously hindered coronary arteries. However, stenting and sidestep methods assisted a few patients with obstinate chest torment, called angina (Liebetrau et al., 2017).

"You would believe that on the off chance that you fix the blockage, the patient will feel good or improve," said Dr. Alice Jacobs, overseer of Cath Lab and Interventional Cardiology at Boston University. The examination, she added, "positively will challenge our clinical reasoning." This is a long way from the primary investigation to propose that stents and sidestep are abused. Yet, past outcomes have not stopped specialists, who have called prior research regarding the matter uncertain and the plan of the preliminaries defective (Liebetrau et al., 2017).

"Past examinations didn't satisfactorily control for hazard factors, similar to LDL cholesterol, that may have influenced results," said Dr. Elliott Antman, a senior doctor at Brigham and Women's Hospital in Boston. "Nor did those preliminaries incorporate the present improved stents, which discharge drugs proposed to keep opened supply routes from shutting once more. With its size and thorough plan, the new investigation, called Ischemia, was expected to settle inquiries concerning the advantages of stents and sidestep." "This is a remarkably significant preliminary," said Dr. Glenn Levine, overseer of cardiovascular consideration at Baylor College of Medicine in Houston. The outcomes will be joined into treatment rules, added Dr. Levine, who sits on the American Heart Association rules board. The members in Ischemia were not encountering a cardiovascular failure, similar to Senator Bernie Sanders, nor did they have blockages of the left principal coronary vein. Two circumstances in which opening conduits with stents can be lifesaving. The patients had limited supply routes that were found with practice pressure tests (Liebetrau et al., 2017).

With 5,179 members followed for three and a half years, Ischemia is the biggest preliminary to address the impact of opening hindered veins in non-emergency circumstances and incorporate the current incredible medication regimens, which specialists allude to as clinical treatment (Liebetrau et al., 2017). Every one of the patients had moderate to severe blockages in coronary veins. Most had some set of experiences of chest torment, albeit one out of three had no chest torment in the prior month enlistment in the investigation—one out of five experienced chest torment in any event once per week (Liebetrau et al., 2017).

All members were routinely guided to stick to clinical treatment. Contingent upon the patient's condition, the treatment differently included high portions of statins and other cholesterol-bringing down drugs, pulse meds, ibuprofen and, for those with heart harm, a medication to moderate the pulse (Liebetrau et al., 2017). Likewise, the individuals who got stents took an incredible enemy of coagulating drugs for a half year to a year. Patients were haphazardly relegated to have clinical treatment alone or mediation and clinical treatment. Of those in the mediation bunch, 3/4 got stents; the others got sidestep a medical procedure (Liebetrau et al., 2017). The quantity of passing among the individuals who had stents or sidestep was 145, contrasted with 144 among the patients who got drug alone. The number of patients who had cardiovascular failures was 276 in the stent and sidestep bunch, contrasted and 314 in the medicine bunch, an immaterial distinction (Liebetrau et al., 2017).

OVERALL QUALITY OF LIFE IN PATIENTS UNDERGOING ANGIOPLASTY

Alongside all the research done on the benefits and issues related to angioplasty, the ultimate test of whether this is an effective treatment is based on clinical trials. Clinical trials are essential as they put research to the test of how much so and whether or not the quality of the patient's lives who undergo angioplasty has changed. There are many different forms of research and epidemiology studies done to test the quality of patients' lives. The different studies conducted are due to testing the differences in outcomes that the varying forms of angioplasty and the disease or illness for which an angioplasty treatment plan is recommended. Types of angioplasty include balloon angioplasty, carotid artery angioplasty, cerebral angioplasty, coronary artery stent angioplasty, laser angioplasty, and percutaneous transluminal angioplasty. Physicians recommend this procedure to patients who suffer from acute coronary syndrome (heart attacks), coronary heart disease, and atherosclerosis. This procedure is also taken into account for less chronic conditions such as treating an abnormal stress test, increasing blood flow to the heart, reducing chest pain (angina), improving blood supply to the heart muscle, and increasing activity for people who have angina.

A five-year longitudinal study was completed by Hueb et al. from 1991 to 1996 to assess the outcomes in patients who have undergone a balloon angioplasty to treat angina alongside single proximal left anterior coronary artery stenosis. In this clinical study, two hundred and fourteen patients were randomly assigned to either receive surgical treatment, angioplasty, or primary medical treatment. After the five-year follow-up, most people who had an occurrence of refractory angina, acute myocardial infarction, or death were the patients who received an angioplasty as treatment (Hueb et al., 1999). Six patients who had surgical treatments showed these symptoms, seventy-two of those who had angioplasty, and seventy-two who had regulatory medical treatment (Hueb et al., 1999).

Eight individuals who underwent angioplasty and medical treatment had to be treated again, but none of those who had surgery needed follow-ups (Hueb et al., 1999). Thus, the study can conclude that to treat angina and single proximal left anterior coronary artery stenosis; a bypass surgery creates the most benefits for the patient instead of an angioplasty. On the contrary, angioplasty was most effective in curing the patient's angina instead of surgery and medical treatment patients.

The complications, issues, and success rates of coronary artery stent angioplasty with individuals affected with myocardial infarction was studied by Perry et al. in 1988. This clinical study was conducted with 224 individuals split into three groups of patients with angina, patients with angina and a history of transmural myocardial infarction, and patients with angina and a history of non-transmural myocardial infarction (Perry et al., 1988). All of these individuals were then treated with a percutaneous transluminal coronary angioplasty. The success rate of percutaneous transluminal coronary angioplasty in the first group was the highest at 90%. The second-highest was group three at 77%, and the lowest success rate was 64% from group two (Perry et al., 1988). This shows that the success rates become lower when treating major illnesses alongside angina than only angina. In addition, the complication of an acute coronary occlusion became present in the highest number of patients in group two (nine individuals), the second-highest amount in group one (seven individuals), and the least amount of patients in group three (four individuals). Thus, the results of this clinical trial indicate that previous history of myocardial infarction becomes a risk factor to be treated with angioplasty since it increases the risk factor for significant complications after treatment (Perry et al., 1988).

Investigating the effects of coronary stent placement angioplasty against balloon angioplasty in the treatment of coronary heart disease (with a specific interest in coronary artery disease) was studied in 1994 by Fischman et al. This study also compared the success rate and repeated prevalence of restenosis (which is a blocked blood artery which can be treated with angioplasty). The study consisted of 410 individuals affected by the symptomatic coronary disease, from which half were treated with balloon angioplasty, and the other half were given a stent angioplasty. The stent angioplasty had an overall greater procedural success rate since the luminal diameter after treatment increased by 1.72mm with a 96.1% rate (Fischman et al., 1994). The balloon angioplasty had a lower but not discrediting effect on patients as a high success rate of 89.6% was observed with the luminal diameter increased by 1.23mm after treatment (Fischman et al., 1994). After a follow-up was done on patients six months after their respective treatments showed that individuals who underwent a stent angioplasty, the luminal diameter was still showing a 1.74mm increase alongside a 31.6% restenosis complication rate. Patients treated with a balloon angioplasty had a luminal diameter steady increase of 1.56mm, as well as a 42.1% restenosis complication rate (Fischman et al., 1994). Significant complications such as death, myocardial infarction, coronary artery bypass surgery, vessel closure, thrombosis, or repeated angioplasty treatment were observed to be higher in the balloon angioplasty group, being 23.8% and lower in the stent angioplasty group, being 19.5% (Fischman et al., 1994). Myocardial ischemia was performed 10.2% in the stent angioplasty group and 15.4% in the balloon angioplasty group (Fischman et al., 1994). Thus, the clinical trial results indicate that either treatment plan is overall effective in treating patients with coronary heart disease. Still, to optimize the success rate and minimize complication rates, a stent angioplasty would produce better results.

Thus far, the quality of life in patients has been studied and explained through clinical and research studies done in the 1900s but to see whether or not these numbers have changed, 2000's research must also be a factor. A longitudinal study conducted by Yamaji et al. from 1989 to 2012 was conducted to study the outcomes of a balloon angioplasty treatment (group one) against metal coronary stenting angioplasty treatment (group two). This study is being conducted as previous research shows that revascularization and restenosis are significant complications that occur after these respective treatments. This trial consisted of 659 patients treated with balloon angioplasty, whereas 405 patients received a metal stent angioplasty (Yamaji et al., 2012). After one year of treatment, death and target lesion thrombosis rates were very similar between group one and two, as they are 44.4% and 45.4%, respectively (Yamaji et al., 2012).

However, group one had higher post-treatment target lesion thrombosis rates than group two after two years (44.6% and 36.0%, respectively). Still, on the contrary group, one had lower rates of such after a four-year follow-up (being 16.3% and 21.4%, respectively). After a ten-year follow-up, lumen loss was higher in group two as observed results state 0.11±0.46mm, whereas in group two it is -0.08±0.45mm (Yamaji et al., 2012). As follows, when treating patients with various diseases and illnesses, a balloon angioplasty would prove to be associated with a higher quality of life and less lumen loss down the line for patients.

Bliley et al. studied how the quality of life in patients changed after receiving a coronary angioplasty in 1993. Forty patients who underwent a percutaneous transluminal coronary angioplasty were observed four to six weeks after treatment (Bliley et al., 1993). The results indicate that the quality of life of the research study participants was delighted with the changes in their life such as considerable improvement in decreased chest pain, decreased cardiac symptoms, increased tolerance of physical activity, increase in the ability to walk long distances, increased time in treadmill tests, and increased overall quality of life (Bliley et al., 1993). In addition to these changes, a significant number of participants also gave up smoking and increased their physical activity rates themselves (Bliley et al., 1993). Thus, receiving a percutaneous transluminal coronary angioplasty significantly changes the quality of life in individuals for the better, and this treatment can be further optimized by follow-ups and a consistently controlled diet post-treatment.

The health-related quality of life improvements after individuals got treated with a stent or standard angioplasty due to their iliac artery occlusive disease was studied in 1999 by Bosch et al. The assessment was done on two hundred and fifty-four patients through an interview-style questionnaire one, three, twelve, and twenty-four months after their respective treatments (Bosch et al., 1999). The results indicate that there is not a very large difference in the improvement between the two treatment plans observed. Thus, one is not overpowering the other in improving the health of the patient overall (Bosch et al., 1999). Improvements seen in patients include physical functioning, fewer role limitations because of their previous disease, and decreased physical pain/sensitivity in stent patients (Bosch et al., 1999). Thus, the researchers can conclude that although the results are the same, those who received a stent angioplasty have slightly more optimal results.

Assessing the health-related quality of life in patients one year after receiving either balloon angioplasty or stent angioplasty to treat their myocardial infarction was studied in 2001 by Rinfret et al. This was done by an administered questionnaire to patients one, six, and twelve months after they were treated in a randomized trial to either receive stent or balloon angioplasty. After the first month's follow-up, patients who received a stent angioplasty reported less bodily pain and sensitivity than the opposing group (Rinfret et al., 2001). After the six-month follow-up, stenting angioplasty still showed more improvements than a balloon angioplasty as there was more improved disease perception and reduced anginal (chest pain) frequencies (Rinfret et al., 2001). After the twelve-month follow-up, there were no significant differences between both groups, as the procedure's benefits were relatively the same. The researchers believe that the slight increase in patients who received a stent angioplasty due to the lower need for repeated ischemia driven target vessel revascularization meant that more patients who provided a balloon angioplasty needed post-treatment (Rinfret et al., 2001). Thus, overall a stent angioplasty would give the best chance of improving the myocardial infarction.

Another research study completed by Pocock et al. in 2000 evaluates the quality of life in patients three years after receiving a coronary angioplasty to treat their angina. A randomized trial was used to randomly assign one thousand and eighteen participants to either the medical treatment group or the percutaneous transluminal coronary angioplasty group. They were split to reduce bias and test if significant differences are seen between the two. To obtain results, the participants answered thirty-six questions based on their self-perceived quality of life after three months, one year, and three years after the respective treatments (Pocock et al., 2000). Overall out of both experimental groups, after one year, 2% of participants had passed away, and 33% had died after three years (Pocock et al., 2000). After three months and one year, the percutaneous transluminal coronary angioplasty group was overpowering the medical treatment group in terms of more significant improvements in physical functioning, vitality, and overall quality of life (these include less breathlessness, less angina, and more excellent treadmill exercise timings). However, after three years, the medical treatment group had a slightly higher quality of life. After three years, the researchers believe that the medical group has better results since 27% of such received more nonrandomized interventions post-treatment (Pocock et al., 2000). Overall, both groups have higher physical functioning, improved social and emotional functioning, less pain/sensitivity, and more excellent mental health. Post one year after treatment, the percutaneous transluminal coronary angioplasty group had a 33% greater health and quality of life, whereas the medical group was 22% (Pocock et al., 2000). Thus, these results indicate that receiving a coronary angioplasty is more effective than medical treatment for those who have angina.

Coronary intervention in the form of angioplasty is often used to treat coronary artery disease. The aftermath of how this procedure affects individuals' health and quality of life is explored by Konstantina et al. in 2009. This article researched all previous studies regarding the effects of coronary angioplasty to compile the knowledge and present the overall epidemiology associated with such (Konstantina et al., 2009). Observations made include the fact that even though coronary angioplasty benefits patients initially, the restenosis rate is high (Konstantina et al., 2009). Furthermore, the effects of this procedure and rate of restenosis are also affected by demographics (such as their sex and family status) and clinical variables (such as their physical state previously if they have a co-existing disease, mental health issues: i.e. depression, and continuing symptoms of angina (Konstantina et al., 2009). Overall, the continuation of healthy habits and lifestyle modifications such as the medications they take, physical exercise rate, and eating a healthy diet are the most important to improve quality of life and keep it that way post-treatment.

After a middle cerebral artery angioplasty to treat severe symptomatic stenosis, the long-term effects and periprocedural stroke rates were studied from 2007 to 2015 by Wang et al. One hundred and ninety-six patients who have severe atherosclerotic stenosis were treated and observed for eight years post-treatment. Improvement in stenosis after thirty days was seen in 98% of patients, and the fatality rate is 2.6% (Wang et al., 2016). The early years in the study have a greater periprocedural stroke rate in participants than the after years as it went from 16.0% to 7.1% (Wang et al., 2016). The mortality rate 6-69 months post the middle cerebral artery angioplasty treatment was reasonably stable at 4.8%, and the regular restenosis rate was 20.4% (Wang et al., 2016). Thus, the research study showed that the success rate is reasonably large. To optimize this treatment plan, patients should be treated with an intracranial angioplasty at a high-volume treatment center with regular follow-ups to avoid complications.

Thus, the various forms of angioplasty (balloon angioplasty, carotid artery angioplasty, cerebral angioplasty, coronary artery stent angioplasty, laser angioplasty, and percutaneous transluminal angioplasty) to treat various types of illnesses and diseases (acute coronary syndrome (heart attacks), coronary heart disease, atherosclerosis, treating an abnormal stress test, increasing blood flow to the heart, reducing chest pain, and improving blood supply to the heart muscle) in patients affect individuals in an overall positive way. The quality of life with health-related issues shows many improvements in those who received a standard coronary angioplasty, percutaneous transluminal coronary angioplasty, stent angioplasty, balloon angioplasty, and cerebral angioplasty. These improvements include decreased chest pain, decreased cardiac symptoms, increased tolerance of physical activity, increase in the ability to walk long distances, increased time in treadmill tests, less bodily pain/sensitivity, less breathlessness, and a lower rate of restenosis. Overall, it can be seen that angioplasty is more effective in treating patients compared to medical treatments or surgery, a coronary stent angioplasty is most effective in those suffering from angina combined with myocardial infarction, and for long term treatment, a balloon angioplasty shows more promising results as opposed to a metal stent coronary angioplasty. As shown, the majority of the results skew in the positive direction. Still, to make sure complications don't arise and that the angioplasty remains intact, it is important for patients post-treatment to follow a balanced healthy diet, practise healthy habits (ex. no smoking), and create a physical activity schedule.

CONTROVERSY OF THE USE OF ANGIOPLASTY

Angioplasty is undoubtedly an essential and innovative procedure. However, due to the risks associated with the process and the numerous life-threatening circumstances in which it may be applied, it remains surrounded by controversy. Differences of opinion about angioplasty can be found between medical professionals and public spaces such as social media and news broadcasters, and government health policy recommendations. Opposing articles supporting and cautioning against angioplasty seem to be published in similar scholarly journals and equal frequency. A 2017 Circulation issue of the American Heart Association published both a topic titled 'Complete Immediate Revascularization of the Patient With ST-Segment–Elevation: Myocardial Infarction Is the New Standard of Care' and an issue titled 'Complete Revascularization of the ST-Segment–Elevation Myocardial Infarction Patient Is Not Yet Proven' regarding angioplasty (Bindhi & Banning, 2017; Oldroyd, 2017). While these two articles both have merit and authority, they demonstrate how divided the scholarly community remains on the procedure. Angioplasty is like any other medical procedure that requires methodical, clinical testing to be approved as a viable treatment in Canada. The effects of this treatment and the associated risks can be proven with well-designed trials and patient participation. So how did a treatment become surrounded by controversy? The answer is as complicated as the procedure itself.

Ever since angioplasty has entered the medical research sphere, there have been doubts about its application in the medical professional community. Angioplasty can be used in hundreds of different treatment strategies to treat hundreds of various pulmonary and cardiological diseases. This broad scope of potential application makes it difficult to apply one judgement to all cases. What may be a dangerous and unnecessarily risky procedure for one patient with one disease, maybe essential and appropriate for another? For example, angioplasty has been used for chronic thromboembolic pulmonary hypertension (CTEPH) as a less-invasive alternative than endarterectomy

(Liebetrau et al., 2017). Due to the risks of artery damage, blood clots, and heart attack, angioplasty has not been suggested for CTEPH patients who can receive an endarterectomy. However, angioplasty treatments have demonstrated promising results, particularly for CTEPH patients deemed inoperable for endarterectomy (Liebetrau et al., 2017). Distinctions with the intent to determine if one strategy is better than another concretely do the least harm possible for the best patient outcome are easier to identify in the CTEPH operable vs inoperable divide; however, that is not always the case.

In some cases, controversy can stem from the fact that there is not enough clinical evidence to determine if one strategy is better than another concretely. For example, acute ischemic stroke (AIS) occurs when a blood clot blocks blood flow to the brain. AIS requires involved and timely treatment, but there are disagreements about the best strategy to remove the blockage (Wilson et al., 2017). Firstly, it is difficult to determine whether to treat the intracranial or extracranial lesions first to restore blood flow and save brain tissue. Some researchers suggest that treating intracranial lesions should be done before extracranial lesions because it saves time for recanalizing the blood vessels. Other researchers suggest that there is better collateralization if the extracranial lesions are treated first. Further to this disagreement, researchers are divided on whether stenting or angioplasty is best for treating extracranial lesions. Those in favour of stenting and angioplasty state that there is a more straightforward and predictable progression of the treatment. In contrast, those in favour of angioplasty alone suggest that the antiplatelet therapy involved with stenting involves a risk of bleeding. Due to these varying approaches, AIS has been treated with thrombectomy alone to push or suck the blockage out of the way, thrombectomy with angioplasty or stenting to support the vessel, and angioplasty followed later by thrombectomy. A study conducted by Wilson et al. attempted to clarify the best course of action; however, they found no statistical difference in extracranial vs intracranial first, nor stenting vs angioplasty by itself (2017). Thus, immediate treatment of AIS involves many decisions, none better than the other as far as the data shows. Even if all of the treatment strategies carry similar risks and effectiveness, this uncertainty serves to fuel the controversy of angioplasty.

A significant argument centring in the controversy of angioplasty is its efficacy compared to pharmaceutical procedures. One of the arenas for these opposing viewpoints is the use of angioplasty versus thrombolysis to treat ST-elevated myocardial infarction (STEMI) heart attacks. A series of studies conducted in Europe examined the differences between angioplasty and thrombolysis treatment based on percent mortality risk (Widimsky, 2010). These studies ultimately found that, based on mortality risk, there was no group of STEMI patients who benefited from thrombolysis than angioplasty. Despite this conclusion, many misconceptions continue to raise questions about whether a pharmaceutical thrombolysis treatment is a better option than angioplasty. The first misconception is that thrombolysis is faster. Studies have previously compared the time between arriving at the treatment location to time receiving either the needle for thrombolysis or the balloon for angioplasty (Tarantini et al., 2010). This is a difficult comparison because it compares receiving the drug to the balloon treatment instead of comparing when the drug becomes effective to the balloon treatment. These comparisons must be drawn to help doctors conclude a particular treatment; however, there must be a consideration for the actual effect on the patient. Another misconception is that thrombolysis is more effective. In terms of opening the artery, thrombolysis has been demonstrated to be 20-60% effective in STEMI patients, whereas angioplasty has been 90% effective in these patients (Widimsky, 2010). Angioplasty may have less of a difference in recovery for low mortality patients than thrombolysis; however, it still stands that the arteries are successfully opened and that the treatments are successful (Widimsky, 2010). Another misconception is that the presentation of coronary thrombi impacts how well angioplasty vs thrombolysis therapy can be used. A study conducted by Tarantini et al. demonstrated that the presentation delay of the coronary thrombosis is a weak predictor of how well either therapy strategy will work (2010). It may be tempting to argue that the quickest displaying treatment is best, but it is essential to keep in mind overall effectiveness. The final misconception about the STEMI treatment comparison is that angioplasty is too difficult to access to bother using instead of thrombolysis. While trials have demonstrated that thrombolysis is an adequate treatment that can be more efficiently delivered to remote regions, the use of thrombolysis while travelling to a centre with angioplasty capability is the best course of action (Widimsky, 2010). Any period of action which might risk someone's life in the name of saving it is likely to come under criticism. As more artery-opening treatments are developed and refined, it is essential to continue to test the efficacy of current practices. The thrombolysis vs angioplasty debate demonstrates that continued methodical and testable criticism is essential to help medical professionals offer the best solutions for their patients.

There are also questions of which pharmaceuticals can be combined with angioplasty to improve results. One such case is the use of beta-block-ers, drugs that reduce adrenaline and slow heart rate, in angioplasty procedures. There have been lower mortality after angioplasty with the use of beta-blockers; however, those results have only been reported for short-term mortality (Faxon, 2004). There is not sufficient evidence for long-term benefits of beta-blocker therapy, although the short-term benefits are adequate to suggest beta-blocker therapy after angioplasty. It is essential to consider that the mechanism of benefit from beta-blocker use has not been elucidated. It is also still unclear if patients receiving primary angioplasty may benefit from oral beta-blocker therapy in the long-term or pre-procedural (Faxon, 2004). Researchers can agree that beta-blockers are beneficial to reduce mortality after angioplasty; however, their specific time frame of application warrants further consideration. A study first published in 2018 confirmed that the use of beta-blockers did not increase mortality or shock in STEMI patients but was unable to guarantee a long-term benefit (Roolvink et al., 2020). There is still a need for further clinical trials to determine the long-term effects of using be-ta-blockers and angioplasty together. A sentiment echoed in many studies examining combining drug therapy with angioplasty. Without these trials and reliable evidence, there is no way to quell conspiracy and controversy concerning the use of these medical methods.

Controversy over medical procedures is not only relegated to the pro-fessional community. A critical case study of angioplasty public opinion and discourse is angioplasty to treat MS in Canada. Multiple sclerosis (MS) is a disease of the nervous system caused by blocked internal veins

(Zamboni et al., 2009). As a result of this proposal, angioplasty has been suggested as a treatment for MS. However, there are doubts in the scientific community about whether MS is caused by the proposed blocked internal veins (Driedger et al., 2018). Furthermore, angioplasty has not been proven to benefit patients with MS (Cardaioli et al., 2016). Despite the lack of proven benefit, coverage on news sources and social media anecdotes have perpetuated the concept of angioplasty as a reliable MS treatment (Snyder et al., 2014). Media communicators such as journalists have the critical job of conveying information in a digestible and nuanced way for public consumption. This can, on occasion, be influenced by the news outlet's political biases as well as the personal biases of the communicators. This communication becomes critical in health service reporting. The reporting language used around procedures can impact how consumers view the medical treatment, regardless of actual risk or benefit. When it comes to medical procedures approved outside of the country, positive language about the treatment can cause medical tourism, where patients travel outside the country to receive treatment (Chang, 2007). As social media has gained traction as an information source, policymakers have even less control over public information about medical treatments. The anonymity of specific social media sites can encourage patients to share sensitive information about their medical travel and treatments. These anecdotes are accessible to other patients without a fact-checking or professional opinion. While these personal experiences can illuminate some facets of the therapy not discussed in the news, social media posts tend to focus on negative experiences with facilities or physicians instead of the actual safety and efficacy of the medicines (Montemurro et al., 2015).

The MS-angioplasty debate took hold in Canada in 2009 when a documentary framed angioplasty as a game-changing treatment for MS (Driedger et al., 2018). This documentary did not explore associated risks in-depth and did not address bias in the anecdotal recovery stories or the evidence. Later, a CTV episode portrayed the treatment positively, exploring the potential benefits to MS patients. There were clips of patients in wheelchairs able to walk after the treatment and quotes about being a possible cure for MS. While there is nothing inherently wrong with discussing the potential of treatment, news networks need to present possible risks; Driedger et al.

credited this CTV episode with inducing Canadian demand for MS-related angioplasty and a jump in medical tourism for the procedure. This was an issue because the little news story impacted public opinion and pressure on policymakers without sufficiently communicating the reality of the treatment, which, at the time, was still largely experimental for treating MS. There was plenty of coverage on the issue following the release of the episode, with 135 stories on the topic in 2011 alone. The trend followed on social media with posts exerting pressure on policymakers to approve angioplasty for MS treatment. The social media posts appeared to sensationalize the issue without displaying neutrality as the news sources did. During this period, the expertise and recommendations of medical scientists and scientific researchers were challenged by patients with MS due to the sensationalizing of the issue by both the news and social media.

In the public sphere, the medical community was criticized for prioritizing professional norms over patient wellbeing and improvements. With the personal and differing experiences with MS, there grew a narrative pitting medical professionals against each other such as neurologists vs vascular surgeons. This was exacerbated by the emphasis of neurologists on proven disease-modifying drugs instead of structural procedures such as angioplasty. This emphasis caused the creation of conspiracies aligning neurologists with big pharma and monetary gains. Further to this, personal anecdotes on social media provided an arena for MS patients seeking this treatment to demand rights to access it under the frame of injustice. The MS patients' willingness to accept the procedure's risks challenged the medical professional's concern over the unproven treatment (Driedger et al., 2018). This controversy reflects a more significant problem in our society today; personal stories are not empirical evidence; however, empirical evidence is only as good as clinical trials. Policymakers, medical professionals, and news networks need to utilize social media to provide the facts about controversial medical treatments such as angioplasty for MS to prevent a narrative of government withholding medical care and extensive pharma control overshadowing the substantial risks and benefits. People with medical conditions should continue to advocate for their right to beneficial treatment, provided they do their best to be educated on the science and not the story.

As with any medical treatment, there are risks and benefits associated with utilizing angioplasty. Angioplasty has been complicated for the medical community to unanimously support or denounce due to the wide variety of diseases and circumstances in which it can be applied. Angioplasty treatment strategies become even more challenging to navigate with a lack of conclusive evidence on their effectiveness than or in combination with different pharmaceutical treatments. The complex nature of medical policy can exacerbate controversy around such procedures by either endorsing them or denying them. Again, a lack of conclusive evidence either in support or against angioplasty across all medical applications has invited criticism of policymakers for either unjustly preventing access to life-saving medical care or for being too blase in allowing a risky procedure. The situation in Canada has become further complicated by personal anecdotes, media sensationalism, and corporate interest. To resolve these issues, researchers need to continue pursuing innovative applications and developments in angioplasty in order to make safer, more effective, and more accessible treatments. Medical professionals need to stay abreast of the advances in research and new information to treat their patients. News outlets need to present the facts in engaging ways to reach their audience without unnecessarily sensationalizing the topic or showing a bias in any particular direction. Finally, the public needs to prioritize credible sources to understand risks and benefits over hearsay when making life-changing medical decisions. In the era of online echo chambers and divisive politics, it is essential to consider both sides of a possible solution so we may all treat and be treated in the best possible way.

ADVANCEMENTS ON RESOURCES LISTED

Since the first percutaneous transluminal balloon angioplasty in 1977, several advances in tools and procedures have been made. This chapter will review the significant developments from 1977 to the present, all while examining the advantages and disadvantages of each new tool. Then, after carefully outlining these, the chapter will look at which limitations have yet to be addressed and future directions in angioplasty tools.

The technique for balloon angioplasty has already been addressed in previous chapters, so it will not be discussed here. Some essential technical refinements have been made in the balloon catheters used for angioplasty (such as decreased radius). Still, arguably the most critical advance in the angioplasty technique was introducing bare-metal stents (Bittl, 1996). Bare metal stents are fenestrated tubes made of stainless steel which scaffold the artery, maintaining its wider diameter following surgery (Bittl, 1996). Previous to the invention of coronary stents, angioplasty results were variable: the procedure did not consistently produce wider artery diameters (Bittl, 1996). Moreover, angioplasty with stents can be used in higher-risk patients who cannot undergo traditional balloon angioplasty (Bittl, 1996). The advantages of stents are so numerous that after the first human implantation of a coronary stent in 1986, the use of balloon angioplasties plateaued (Bittl, 1996).

The first type of stent to be employed was termed a bare-metal stent since it is made simply of a bare-metal platform. Among bare-metal stents, several different designs have been created. In general, an optimal stent has the following features: a range of possible diameters and lengths, flexibility, a thin stent material and high radiopacity to allow for precise positioning of the stent (Ozaki et al., 1996). Depending on the specific artery and patient, different stent designs may be optimal (Ozaki et al., 1996). In general, one can distinguish bare-metal stents into two classes: closed-cell and open-cell (Chae et al., 2016). There is very little space between adjacent struts in closed-cell stents, resulting in a dense, rigid metallic mesh (Chae et al., 2016). In contrast, open-cell stents have much more space between struts, giving them a much more flexible structure (Chae et al., 2016). Due to their differences in flexibility, closed-cell stents are most appropriate for straight arterial or venous regions, while open-cell stents are used for kinked regions (Chae et al., 2016).

So far, this chapter has praised bare-metal stents for their advantages over traditional balloon angioplasties. Conversely, there are several limitations associated with bare-metal stents. A medical device composed of metal is inherently incompatible with the blood vessels (Jeewandara et al., 2014). In the long term, this incompatibility can cause chronic inflammation and trigger thrombosis (blood clot formation) (Jeewandara et al., 2014). Thrombosis is the major complication associated with bare-metal stents; it occurs in up to 24% of angioplasties with bare-metal stents if concurrent antiplatelet therapy is not used (Jeewandara et al., 2014). Thrombosis is also incredibly dangerous: it may cause heart attacks or death (Jeewandara et al., 2014). Another complication associated with bare-metal stents is restenosis, in which the artery narrows following angioplasty (Jeewandara et al., 2014). Restenosis occurs due to an overzealous immune response which promotes hyper-growth of smooth muscle cells on the stent platform (Jeewandara et al., 2014).

A revolutionary change to the classic bare metal stent design was the engineering of drug-eluting stents capable of delivering drugs directly to the site of surgery following the procedure (Serruys et al., 1996). Before this development, patients had to follow an anticoagulant drug regimen after their surgeries to prevent subacute thrombosis (Bittl, 1996). However, the anticoagulant drug regimen—which at the time was the first-line preventative treatment for thrombosis—often caused dangerous bleeding and also did not necessarily prevent subacute thrombotic occlusion from occurring (Bittl, 1996). Moreover, first, dangerous statistics outlined the need for a new preventative treatment: in 3.5% of cases, the artery became partially occluded, in 13.9%, bleeding complications occurred, and the average in-hospital stay post-surgery—8.3 days—was unsatisfactory (Serruys et al., 1996). All of these reasons explain why the development of drug-eluting stents (DESs) was so revolutionary.

The prototype of this type of stent was the heparin-coated stent (Bittl, 1996). This type of stent has the drug heparin permanently bound, which is an anticoagulant that prevents the formation of blood clots (Serruys et al., 1996). The bound heparin interacts with molecules and enzymes in the circulating blood, allowing it to exert its anticoagulant effects (Serruys et al., 1996). Heparin acts via three mechanisms to prevent the formation of blood clots (Serruys et al., 1996). First, it prevents the body from initiating a cascade of events that trigger blood coagulation (thickening) (Serruys et al., 1996). Second, heparin prevents enzymes from the cascade which have already been activated from further acting to promote clot formation (Serruys et al., 1996). Finally, heparin prevents blood cells called platelets from adhering to the stent (Serruys et al., 1996). Since platelet adhesion is an essential step in forming blood clots, this mechanistic step is essential in heparin's action against thrombotic occlusion.

While it may seem that creating heparin-coated stents would be as simple as coating a stent with heparin, this is not the case (Emanuelsson et al., 1994). When developing intravascular devices—devices that enter blood vessels—the designers must consider the device's compatibility with the blood (Emanuelsson et al., 1994). For example, when a foreign surface comes in contact with the blood, proteins and other blood components will be deposited onto the surface (Emanuelsson et al., 1994). At the same time, blood coagulation will be initiated, and a response by the immune system will be activated (Emanuelsson et al., 1994). All three of these events are undesirable, as they can lead to clot formation and narrowing of the blood vessel in question (Emanuelsson et al., 1994). For this reason, the stent must be microscopically smooth and made chemically unreactive by a technique known as electropolishing (Serruys et al., 1996). In addition, the stent must be coated with substances that resist clot formation, such as hydrogels or polyurethanes (Serruys et al., 1996).

Another question that must be considered in developing heparin-coated stents is: how do we attach heparin to the stent? The problem with simply coating the stent with a heparin layer is that it is impossible to control the rate of release of the drug into circulation (Serruys et al., 1996). Two possible options to avoid this problem, including incorporating heparin into a polymer that coats the stent (Serruys et al., 1996). In the first option, the heparin is transiently incorporated into the polymer. The polymer makes it possible to control the rate at which heparin is released from the polymer and enters the bloodstream (Serruys et al., 1996). In the second option, the heparin is permanently enmeshed in the polymer; but, the portion of heparin that reacts with plasma proteins is exposed (Serruys et al., 1996). This option, called surface-grafted heparin, was only made possible once researchers developed a method of attaching heparin to the polymer without modifying the portion of heparin responsible for its anticoagulant activity (Serruys et al., 1996).

However, while the theory supporting heparin-coated stents is intense, studies comparing heparin-coated and bare-metal stents in terms of adverse health outcomes are conflicting. On the one hand, some studies show a reduction in adverse health outcomes (Moer et al., 2001; Krajewski et al., 2015). For example, Krajewski and colleagues found that activation of platelet adhesion and blood coagulation (which are both required for blood clot formation) was lower with heparin-coated as opposed to bare metal stents; however, it is worth noting that this study was performed in vitro—outside the body (Krajewski et al., 2015). Another study in 2004 with 1288 patients found that rates of blood clot formation and sudden cardiac death were lower for heparin-coated than bare-metal stents (Aravamuthan et al., 2004).

But several studies have found no difference between heparin-coated and bare-metal stents in terms of rates of blood clot formation, heart attacks, death and restenosis (Wöhrle et al., 2001; Semiz et al., 2003; Mehran et al., 2005). While there are mixed findings with regards to the benefits of heparin-coated as compared to bare metal stents, a study with 145 patients found that heparin-coated stents were at least better than traditional balloon angioplasty in terms of increased blood vessel diameter and a lower rate of adverse health outcomes such as heart attack, indicating that some technological progress was made with their invention (Moer et al., 2001). Moreover, heparin-coated stents are very safe and well-tolerated by patients, and there is also evidence to suggest that covered stents, in general, are safer than bare-metal stents (Serruys et al., 1996; Mwipatayi et al., 2011). The development of heparin stents also paved the way for other types of drug-eluting stents (DESs) to be created.

In general, after the initial development of the heparin-coated stent, the creation of DESs has been divided into three generations. The design of first-generation DESs is very similar to that of the initial heparin proto-type. They consist of a metallic stent coated in a polymer combined with the drug of choice (Simard et al., 2014). Typically, the metal platform is made of stainless steel for the first generation design (Simard et al., 2014). One notable example is the sirolimus-eluting stent (SES). SESs release sirolimus, an immunosuppressive drug that prevents cell growth (Simard et al., 2014). By suppressing the immune system, sirolimus prevents un-desirable inflammation at the site of angioplasty; in addition, it prevents cells from replicating by halting cell cycle progression (Simard et al., 2014). Cell growth must be initially presented at the stent site to prevent a phenomenon known as in-stent restenosis (ISR), where the blood vessel narrows due to cells growing on the stent (Simard et al., 2014). Since the purpose of angioplasty is to widen the artery, ISR is an undesirable event. By stopping cell cycle progression and suppressing the immune system, sirolimus should reduce adverse health outcomes.

The other type of first-generation DES developed is the paclitaxel-eluting stent (PES). Like sirolimus, paclitaxel also prevents cell growth, in this case by stabilizing microtubules (Simard et al., 2014). Microtubules are essentially long molecular branches required to move chromosomes and stretch the cell during cell replication (mitosis). To fulfill this role, they must be very unstable by constantly growing or shrinking. By stabilizing microtubules, paclitaxel prevents cell replication, which lowers the chance of in-stent restenosis (Simard et al., 2014).

First-generation PESs and SESs are very similar in design, and they share es-sential advantages compared to bare metal or heparin-coated stents. First-gen-eration DESs are highly successful in that they considerably reduced the rate of ISR (vessel narrowing) and target vessel revascularization (TVR), which is when vessel narrowing is so severe that a vessel-widening procedure must be repeated (Emst and Bulum, 2014). However, there are questions about its safety in stent thrombosis (ST), where a blood clot forms on the stent, blocking blood flow. Varenhorst and colleagues report that post-angioplasty first-generation DESs show lower ST rates for the first year, but beyond this time, bare-metal stents are associated with lower ST (Varenhorst et al., 2018). In particular, it was found that the thickness of the DESs is indirectly related to the formation of ST (Whitbeck and Applegate, 2013).

Also, the polymers used in first-generation DESs are not optimally biocompatible (Ernst and Bulum, 2014). Human autopsies of angioplasty patients with first-generation DESs identified several concerns with the devices; these concerns include chronic inflammation in the blood vessel walls, delayed arterial healing following stent implantation, and accelerated formation of new atherosclerotic plaques (Ernst and Bulum, 2014). The polymers from first-generation DESs may also cause several mechanical issues within the stent, such as the polymer becoming detached from the metal base or the inability of the stent to expand properly (Ernst and Bulum, 2014).

In response to accumulating concerns, the second generation of DESs was born. During the second generation, PESs and SESs were abandoned entirely due to concerns about clot formation (Whitbeck and Applegate, 2013). Instead, zotarolimus- and everolimus-eluting stents (ZESs and EESs, respectively) were developed, with slightly differing stent designs (Simard et al., 2014). The ZES design features a thinner metal platform to minimize clot formation, which is made possible by using cobalt-chromium instead of stainless steel (Simard et al., 2014; Tantawy, 2014). It also features a new phosphorylcholine polymer coating; this coating mimics the chemical structure of the lipid cell membrane, which makes it more biocompatible and hence minimizes inflammation occurring due to immune reaction (Simard et al., 2014). In addition, the phosphorylcholine polymer also reduces the time for drug release (Simard et al., 2014). This means that zotarolimus is present immediately after surgery to suppress the immune system, but not so late afterwards that it interferes with arterial repair (Simard et al., 2014). In terms of zotarolimus itself, it has similar immunosuppressive properties to sirolimus. But compared to sirolimus, it is more lipophilic (attracted to lipids), which makes the drug more attracted to the vessel walls than the blood—effectively keeping the medicine at the stent site as opposed to travelling within the circulation (Simard et al., 2014).

EESs share a similar chromium cobalt platform design but differ in terms of the polymer used (Whitbeck and Applegate, 2013). They are composed of a copolymer with vinylidene fluoride and hexafluoropropylene (Whitbeck and Applegate, 2013). This copolymer has outstanding biocompatibility and stability in the body; it also can deliver everolimus at a lower dose than the first-generation polymers, an essential factor in preventing drug toxicity (Whitback and Applegate, 2013). Like zotarolimus, everolimus is an analogue of sirolimus with similar immunosuppressive properties but higher lipophilicity (Allocco et al., 2011).

Later during the second generation of development, the durable polymers of the first and early second generation were replaced with bioresorbable polymers, which dissolve over time (Ernst and Bulum, 2014). One such example is a polylactic acid polymer that dissolves thoroughly after six to nine months, used in combination with a cobalt-chromium platform (Ernst and Bulum, 2014). After the polymer has dissolved, the remaining device is essentially equivalent to a bare-metal stent (Ernst and Bulum, 2014). This new polymer was created to avoid the higher stent thrombosis (ST) rate of DESs than bare-metal stents while still maintaining the drug-eluting capacity and lower restenosis rate (vessel narrowing) of DESs.

However, some studies have found that rates of ST and target vessel revascularization (TVR; where the vessel narrows considerably) are not significantly different between stents with durable compared to bioresorbable polymers (Ahmed et al., 2011). Nevertheless, the development of biopolymer-based DES was an important step leading to the third generation of DESs: bioabsorbable drug-eluting vascular scaffolds (BVS). BVSs are entirely bioabsorbable—both the polymer and the scaffold (Ernst and Bulum, 2014). The device provides temporary support and integrity to the blood vessel following angioplasty but dissolves after it is no longer needed (Ernst and Bulum, 2014). They are intended to provide temporary support to the vessel as well as drug delivery while avoiding the complications of long-term metal stents such as blood clot formation and chronic inflammation, among others (Ernst and Bulum, 2014). In addition, advantages associated with BVSs instead of bare metal stents include the possibility of later revascularization interventions in the area and the ability to non-invasively image the area with CT or MRI (Ernst and Bulum, 2014).

But, BVSs are still in their infancy, and as such, several issues have yet to be resolved. Unlike metals, the properties of the same polymer can vary per batch and manufacturer and are based on processing and stocking conditions (Sharkawi et al., 2007). These differences can result in varying biocompatibility and unpredictable reactions within the body (Sharkawi et al., 2007). Results from studies on BVSs can also fluctuate based on these variables, making it difficult to synthesize a consistent body of research on them (Sharkawi et al., 2007). In general, the research is still inconclusive about whether BVSs are safer or more effective than second-generation DESs, but some research has indicated that they are a feasible option in a wide spectrum of patients (Azzalini et al., 2016; Jaguszewski et al., 2015). More research is needed to develop this new and emerging technology.

Through this chapter, the history of angioplasty was explored through the lens of evolving stent technologies. The technology has evolved in leaps and bounds since the first angioplasty in 1977 and the implantation of the first bare-metal stent in 1986. It is hard to believe that almost three generations of drug-eluting stents have passed in such a short period. Nevertheless, we are in an exciting era of biomedical engineering history: the third generation of DESs is still in its infancy. There are many more technically brilliant designs to be witnessed.

FUTURE PROSPECTS OF ANGIOPLASTY

INTRODUCTION

This chapter approaches the prospects of angioplasty using two conceptual vantage points: firstly, the perspective stemming from disease prevention and, secondly, the treatment improvement perspective. Disease prevention is a remarkably underserved topic in health care in general (perhaps due to the inherent, and often nefarious, financial incentives of the pharmaceutical industry. There is little money to be had in disease prevention, but disease treatment, on the other hand, is a highly profitable industry. For this reason, not much research exists in preventing coronary artery disease compared to the perfection of the angioplasty procedure. From the accessible information gathered for this chapter, two warring factors prevent and promote coronary artery disease in turn. These factors, identified further in subsequent sections, include adopting a plant-based diet and the social determinants of health that are furthered by increasing income inequality in most developed countries (Tuso et al., 2015) (Kondro, 2002). While the increasing number of people who identify as vegan may reduce the rate of incidence of coronary artery disease in industrialized nations, this trend could be offset by the rising income inequality, as it has been demonstrated that poverty is correlated with poor health outcomes (especially in the case of obesity-related illnesses such as coronary artery disease) (Waitzman & Smith, 1998).

The effectiveness of the angioplasty procedure has improved over time due to rigorous scientific trial and error (Chandrakant & Nanjappa 2017). Through this trial and error method, scientists have moved from attempting to merely understand the circulatory system to innovate new methods of drug administration to prevent restenosis post-angioplasty procedure. Improvements mentioned in this chapter include the use of robotics (Smilowitz & Weisz, 2012), the use of bio-degradable stents (Di Mario et al., 2015), IIb/IIIa inhibitors (Oomman & Ramachandran, 2001) (De Luca et al., 2015), and the 'rendezvous technique'(Nihei et al., 2017). Each of these improvements could pave the future of the angioplasty procedure.

The future of the angioplasty procedure is uncertain. It is inherently difficult, if not impossible, to predict future scientific advancements. Who among Isaac Newton could have predicted his discovery of gravity, for instance? The aims of the society are, however, quite specific. The goal of scientists is to reduce human suffering incurred by illness and injury, a sentiment echoed by the Hippocratic oath. This alone can bring some hope that in the future, the angioplasty procedure will be improved if not made obsolete by disease prevention.

DISEASE PREVENTION TO CONTRIBUTE TO THE OBSOLESCENCE ANGIOPLASTY PROCEDURES

Coronary artery disease is the leading cause of death in the United States (Rana et al., 2020). The importance of improving angioplasty procedures to prevent these deaths is equalled by the need to avoid the illness from occurring in the first place. Coronary artery disease is an obesity-related illness, meaning that diet and exercise are two important factors contributing to the rates at which this illness occurs. Specifically, a plant-based diet that is low in cholesterol, fat and sodium is correlated with a lower rate of incidences of coronary artery disease (Tuso et al., 2015). One study found that the patients diagnosed with heart disease and who followed a plant-based diet had a reduced likelihood of experiencing angina episodes (Tuso et al., 2015). Another study found that a plant-based diet was correlated with a 73% reduction in the likelihood of cardiac events (de Lorgeril et al., 1999). In addition, patients who adopt a plant-based diet have lower LDL levels and fewer instances of microinflammation (Tuso et al., 2015). Even the Journal of the American Heart Association has conducted research demonstrating the correlation between adopting a plant-based diet and a reduction in general mortality and cardiovascular morbidity (Kim et al., 2019). For various reasons, including environmental, ethical, and health, the number of people who identify as vegans has been rapidly increasing in industrialized nations (Janssen et al., 2016).

The effect of this increase in plant-based persons could correspond with a subsequent decrease in the number of people who have coronary artery disease and require an angioplasty procedure to treat it. This would enable individuals to avoid the ailments that need them to go under the knife and endure costs to their health and pockets. Disease prevention is a crucial ingredient in public health policies. It solves disease at the source rather than applying a procedural bandage that cannot reverse the illness itself, coronary artery disease. Therefore, the future of angioplasty may, thankfully, be a reduction in the number of operations needing to be performed as a result of the betterment of overall health, which is promoted by a plant-based, nutrient-dense diet.

INCREASING INCOME INEQUALITY MAY RESULT IN A CORRESPONDING INCREASE IN CORONARY ARTERY DISEASE AND AN INCREASED DEMAND FOR ANGIOPLASTY PROCEDURES

This decrease in the need for angioplasty procedures due to an increase in adoptions of plant-based diets may be offset by an increase in income inequality, as poverty is a risk factor in determining the health outcomes of individuals (especially in instances of obesity-related illnesses such as coronary artery disease). One Canadian study found that the number one predictor for heart disease is poverty (Kondro, 2002). Dennis Raphael, a professor from York University, Canada, has said that public health policy that focuses on reducing rates of obesity only serves the purpose of blaming the poor for their health outcomes (Kondro, 2002). Material deprivation, a lack of safe, affordable and nourishing food and water, educational disparities and a lack of recreational opportunities make it more likely that those living in low-income communities have an increased need for angioplasty procedures due to higher rates of coronary artery disease (Kondro, 2002).

The increase in income inequality in the United States has been accompanied by a physical separation between the rich and poor in urban areas. Access to healthy foods is not equal in all geographic regions, which has contributed to the disparities in health outcomes attributed to income inequality (Waitzman & Smith, 1998). If income inequality continues to increase, we may see an increased demand for angioplasty procedures as rates of coronary artery disease increase. This does not need to be the case, however. Professor Dennis Raphael has suggested a number of ways in which poverty can be reduced. Higher unemployment/welfare insurance, the creation of a national and affordable child care program, better safeguarding against discrimination and the increased dedication in the way of gender parity, can, interestingly, reduce instances of people with coronary artery disease from needing an angioplasty procedure or from being diagnosed with the illness at all (Kondro, 2002).

UTILIZATION OF ROBOTICS IN CONDUCTING ANGIOPLASTY PROCEDURES

In the first-ever in-person PCI procedure, which was conducted using robotic-assisted technology, the total technical success rate was 97.9% (Smilowitz & Weisz, 2012). In addition, robotic technology will significantly reduce hazards associated with the angioplasty procedure. For instance, robotic technology can reduce the operator's radiation exposure and prevent them from incurring orthopedic or musculoskeletal injuries (Smilowitz & Weisz, 2012). Operators are, of course, not the only ones who stand to benefit from the utilization of robotics in angioplasty procedures; patients are also likely to receive a better quality of care. Robotic technology also reduces radiation exposure for patients and allows for greater mechanical precision in stent placement (Smilowitz & Weisz, 2012). Professor Sabatier of Caen University Hospital has stated that given that Europe has seen its first in-person PCI stent placement procedure on an animal, the next step would be to utilize this groundbreaking new technology on a human subject (Nicholls, 2021).

Professor Eric Durand and Professor Rémi Sabatier successfully implanted a stent using an animal test subject, a pig. Communication between Sabatier and Durand was also facilitated using technology. The two even further complicated the procedure to rigorously test the robotic assistance, by recrossing the stent struts in the septal branch (Nicholls, 2021). As the procedure was successful, the future of angioplasty, and many other surgical procedures, may be changed through the instrumentalization of robotic assistance.

WEIGHING THE BENEFITS OF BIODEGRADABLE VERSUS NON-BIODEGRADABLE STENTS AND THE PREVENTION OF RESTENOSIS

Biodegradable stents have been proposed as an alternative to the metal stents typically utilized by doctors in the performance of angioplasty procedures. Biodegradable stents are, in theory, preferable to metal ones, given the risk of thrombosis (blood clotting) is elevated by having a foreign object permanently within the artery (Di Mario et al., 2015). Researchers found that 16% of patients who received a biodegradable had further angina episodes, as opposed to 26% of the metal stent recipients experiencing angina post-procedure. This proposes a marketable, statistically significant difference in the future life prospects of patients who receive biodegradable, as opposed to conventional metal, stents (Di Mario et al., 2015). Di Mario et al. rightfully point out that much more research is needed to uncover the benefits of biodegradable stents truly. In the absence of such megatrials to confirm the veracity of smaller studies' claims, doctors and patients must consider the incremental, modest benefits that a biodegradable stent could have for the patient's future health (Di Mario et al., 2015).

On the other hand, Chandrakant and Nanjappa argue that the use of biodegradable stents has been somewhat underwhelming in its practical use on the operating table (Chandrakant & Nanjappa 2017). From William Harvey's description of circulation in 1628 to the approval of the first biodegradable stent in 2011, the evolution of the coronary angioplasty procedure has been marked by trial and error. We have come a long way through this process since the simple balloon angioplasty of 1979 (Chandrakant & Nanjappa 2017). In analyzing the history of the angioplasty procedure, Chandrakant and Nanjappa leave off their discussion not on the promising future of biodegradable stents but on the current problem needing to be solved of the delivery of medications to reduce the possibility of the patient experiencing restenosis (the narrowing of a blood vessel resulting in the restriction of blood flow) after the placement of the stent. The early trials of the oral administration of medications preventing restenosis were not adequate. Catheter-based drug administration also proved ineffective; doctors tried coating the stent in medication instead, which proved to be a more successful method of delivery to prevent restenosis (Chandrakant & Nanjappa 2017). Chandrakant and Nanjappa end off their article by stating, "We would like to conclude with: 'Let the hands which intervene be rested on shoulders with responsibility and respect for it with feet firmly on the ground aided by judiciousness and a balance of mind which would dictate the do's and don'ts and not see the person on cath lab table as an experimental tool; let our actions be guided by compassion and patient safety.'"

USE OF IIB/IIIA INHIBITORS

The use of antiplatelet agents (glycoprotein IIb/IIIa inhibitors) may be an additional method to restore blood flow to/from the heart when accompanied with a primary angioplasty procedure (Oomman & Ramachandran, 2001). These inhibitors may increase the likelihood of survival for high-risk patients and prevent stent thrombosis (blood clotting) (De Luca et al., 2015). When administered early on, IIb/IIIa inhibitors may prevent complications from occurring (impaired reperfusion, the successful flow of blood). For this reason, De Luca et al. are supportive of the implementation of the IIb/IIIa inhibitor strategy. The future of angioplasty procedures may involve a less invasive treatment, such as the introduction of IIb/IIIa inhibitors, to increase the procedure's effectiveness.

THE IMPACT OF COVID 19 ON PATIENTS

Postponed appointments to screen for and treat coronary artery disease will have a profound and ongoing impact on patients' health (Nicholls, 2021). As doctors trudge through the backlog in procedures, we may see an increase in angioplasty procedures in the immediate future. Additionally, the delay in treatment may very well have had a significant adverse effect on patients who have not yet received this procedure. When these angioplasty procedures do occur, the illness may have progressed and worsened, such that the survival of the patients will be made less likely. Given that coronary artery disease is already such a deadly illness, these complications could prove fatal to many afflicted individuals.

ADDITIONAL INTRACORONARY TECHNIQUES

Many additional intracoronary techniques have been identified as having the potential to improve upon the established coronary angiographic procedures. Angioplasty procedures are made more difficult and consequently more hazardous due to vessel tears obscuring the operator's view of the vessel walls (Emanuelsson, 1995). Intravascular ultrasounds, an emerging new technology, may assist operators in understanding these lesions. Angioscopy, which can be performed during an angioplasty procedure, is also beneficial for an increased ability to delineate the vessel. An angioscopy is even better than intravascular ultrasounds for identifying intracoronary thrombi, a blockage of the vessel due to plaque rupture, though it cannot find longitude and depth of vessel damage (Emanuelsson, 1995). An angioscopy can also be used to identify the type of plaque buildup. Yellow plaques tend to be more common when the patient suffers from a recent myocardial infarction or unstable angina. White plaques buildup, on the other hand, is associated with more stable angina. However, it is an unfortunate disadvantage that angioscopy requires an exchange in catheters Emanuelsson, 1995). Emanuelsson holds that despite this disadvantage, angioscopy is still promising due to its assistance in maneuvering precise stent placement.

Nihei et al. also describe a "Rendevous technique" in which chronic total occlusion (blockage) is reminded using bidirectional wiring. The rendezvous technique may improve reperfusion (Nihei et al., 2017). This technique can be used for peripheral and well as coronary chronic total occlusion lesions, thanks to new emerging technologies. This technique will be a viable, primary option for operators of the angioplasty procedure in the future (Nihei et al., 2017).

CONCLUSION

The future of angioplasty is uncertain yet of grave importance given the astronomical death rates due to coronary artery disease in industrialized nations. This chapter explored the value of preventative lifestyles and corrective treatments mitigating the development and symptoms of coronary artery disease. The future of angioplasty will rely on scientific advancements made in perfecting the angioplasty procedure. Still, it will also depend on the general health and wellbeing of people in industrialized nations. In discussing the future possibilities of angioplasty, we must question what we truly want to advance, human health or scientific achievements. We already understand what it takes to prevent coronary artery disease- diet and lifestyle are fundamental in this vein of thought. Though there is much debate regarding the angioplasty procedure, it has been established that a healthy lifestyle involves plenty of fruits and vegetables, a reasonable exercise regimen and an ability to keep stress levels under control. In addition, the unequal social conditions that cause health disparities between low and high-income communities should be considered more carefully by scientists and public health legislators. There are several ways in which the angioplasty procedure can be perfected, allowing more lives to be saved. A few avenues of improvement include the prevention of restenosis through medication (Chandrakant & Nanjappa 2017), the use of antiplatelet agents (Oomman & Ramachandran, 2001), and angioscopy and intravascular ultrasounds (Emanuelsson, 1995).

WORKS CITED

Angioplasty and Stent Placement for the Heart. (n.d.). Retrieved May 11, 2021, from https://www.hopkinsmedicine.org/health/treatment-tests-and-therapies/angioplasty-and-stent-placement-for-the-heart

Ahmed, T. A. N., Bergheanu, S. C., Stijnen, T., Plevier, J. W. M., Quax, P. H. A., & Jukema, J. W. (2011). Clinical performance of drug-eluting stents with biodegradable polymeric coating: A meta-analysis and systematic review. In *EuroIntervention* (Vol. 7, Issue 4, pp. 505–516). EuroIntervention.
DOI: 10.4244/EIJV7I4A81

Allocco, D. J., Joshi, A. A., & Dawkins, K. D. (2011). Everolimus-eluting stents: Update on current clinical studies. In *Medical Devices: Evidence and Research* (Vol. 4, Issue 1, pp. 91–98). Dove Press.
DOI: 10.2147/MDER.S22043

Azzalini, L., Giustino, G., Ojeda, S., Serra, A., la Manna, A., Ly, H. Q., Bellini, B., Benincasa, S., Chavarría, J., Gheorghe, L. L., Longo, G., Miccichè, E., D'Agosta, G., Picard, F., Pan, M., Tamburino, C., Latib, A., Carlino, M., Chieffo, A., & Colombo, A. (2016). Procedural and Long-Term Outcomes of Bioresorbable Scaffolds Versus Drug-Eluting Stents in Chronic Total Occlusions. *Circulation: Cardiovascular Interventions*, 9(10).
DOI: 10.1161/CIRCINTERVENTIONS.116.004284

Barton M, Grüntzig J, Husmann M, Rösch J. (2014). Balloon Angioplasty - The Legacy of Andreas Grüntzig, M.D. (1939-1985). Front Cardiovasc Med. 2014;1:15.
DOI:10.3389/fcvm.2014.00015

Bayar, R. (2013). High technology in medicine: Lesson from cardiovascular innovations and future perspective. *Rambam Maimonides Medical Journal*, 4(2), e0009.
DOI: 10.5041/RMMJ.10109

Bhimji, S., & Cunha, J. P. (2019). Peripheral Vascular Disease (PVD) Medical Definition, Signs & Symptoms. EMedicineHealth. https://www.emedicinehealth.com/peripheral_vascular_disease/article_em.htm

Bhindi, R., & Banning, A. P. (2017). Not So Fast: Complete Revascularization of the ST-Segment–Elevation Myocardial Infarction Patient Is Not Yet Proven. *Circulation*, 135(17), 1574-1576.
DOI: 10.1161/CIRCULATIONAHA.116.025266

Bittl, J. A. (1996). Advances in Coronary Angioplasty. *New England Journal of Medicine, 335*(17), 1290–1302.
DOI: 10.1056/nejm199610243351707

Bliley, A.V., & Ferrans, C.E. (1993). Quality of life after coronary angioplasty. *Heart and Lung Journal, 2*(3), 193-9.
DOI: 10.1016/s0735-1097(99)00637-3

Bosch, J.L., Graaf, Y., & Hunink, M.G. (1999). Health-related quality of life after angioplasty and stent placement in patients with iliac artery occlusive disease: results of a randomized controlled clinical trial. *Journal of Circulation, 99*(24), 3155-60.
DOI: 10.1161/01.cir.99.24.3155

Cardaioli, G., Di Filippo, M., Bianchi, A., Eusebi, P., Di Gregorio, M., Gaetani, L., Gallina, A., Calabresi, P., & Sarchielli, P. (2016). Extracranial venous drainage pattern in multiple sclerosis and healthy controls: Application of the 2011 diagnostic criteria for chronic cerebrospinal venous insufficiency. *European neurology, 76*(1-2) 62-68.
DOI: 10.1159/000445540

Cardiologist, A. (2019, July 31). Recent Advances in Coronary Angioplasty. *Apollo Hospitals Blog.* https://healthlibrary.askapollo.com/recent-advances-in-coronary-angioplasty/

Chandrakant, N & Nanjappa, V. (2017). Coronary angioplasty: Back to the future. *Journal of the Practice of Cardiovascular Sciences.* 3. 44
DOI:10.4103/jpcs.jpcs_1_17

Chang, C. T. (2007). Interactive effects of message framing, product perceived risk, and mood—The case of travel healthcare product advertising. *Journal of Advertising Research, 47*(1), 51-65.
DOI: 10.2501/S0021849907070067

Chhabra L, Zain MA, Siddiqui WJ. Angioplasty. [Updated 2020 Aug 10]. In: StatPearls [Internet]. Treasure Island (FL): StatPearls Publishing; 2021 Jan-. Available from: https://www.ncbi.nlm.nih.gov/books/NBK499894/

Coronary Artery Disease: Causes, Symptoms, Diagnosis & Treatments. (n.d.). Cleveland Clinic. https://my.clevelandclinic.org/health/diseases/16898-coronary-artery-disease

De Lorgeril M, Salen P, Martin JL, Monjaud I, Delaye J, Mamelle N. (1999) Mediterranean diet, traditional risk factors, and the rate of cardiovascular complications after myocardial infarction: final report of the Lyon Diet Heart Study. *Circulation* Feb;99(6):779–85.
DOI: 10.1161/01.CIR.99.6.779

De Luca, G. , Savonitto, S. , van't Hof, A. W. & Suryapranata, H. (2015). Platelet GP IIb-IIIa Receptor Antagonists in Primary Angioplasty: Back to the Future. *Drugs,*

75(11), 1229–1253.
DOI: 10.1007/s40265-015-0425-7.

Di Mario, C., & Caiazzo, G. (2015). Biodegradable stents: the golden future of angioplasty? *The Lancet (British Edition), 385*(9962), 10–12.
DOI:10.1016/S0140-6736(14)61636-6

Driedger, S. M., Dassah, E., & Marrie, R. A. (2018). Contesting Medical Miracles: A Collective Action Framing Analysis of CCSVI and Venous Angioplasty ("Liberation Therapy") for People With Multiple Sclerosis in News and Social Media. *Science Communication, 40*(4), 469-498.
DOI: 10.1177%2F1075547018781958

Dunham, E. K., & Herter, C. A. (1907). THE COLLECTED WORKS OF CARL WEIGERT. *Journal of the American Medical Association, 48*(5), 412-415.

Eldmarany, H., Khalefa, S. & El Bahaey, A. (2020). Drug-coated balloon angioplasty for failing arteriovenous fistulae: Feasibility and short-term outcomes. *The Egyptian Journal of Surgery, 39*: 932-938.
DOI:10.4103/ejs.ejs_118_20

Emanuelsson, H., van der Giessen, W. J., & Serruys, P. W. (1994). Benestent II: Back to the Future. *Journal of Interventional Cardiology, 7*(6), 587–592.
DOI: 10.1111/j.1540-8183.1994.tb00500.x

Ernst, A., & Bulum, J. (2014). New Generations of Drug-eluting Stents-A Brief Review. *EMJ Interventional Cardiology, 1*(1), 100–106.

Gaziano T, Reddy KS, Paccaud F, et al. Cardiovascular Disease. In: Jamison DT, Breman JG, Measham AR, et al. (2006). Chapter 33. Cardiovascular Disease. *Disease Control Priorities in Developing Countries (2nd Edition),* 645–662.
DOI:10.1596/978-0-8213-6179-5/chpt-33

Gupta, V., Aravamuthan, B. R., Baskerville, S., Smith, S. K., Gupta, V., Lauer, M. A., & Fischell, T. A. (2004). Reduction of subacute stent thrombosis (SAT) using heparin-coated stents in a large-scale, "real world" registry. *Journal of Invasive Cardiology, 16*(6), 304–310. PMID: 15155999

Faxon, D. P. (2004). Beta-blocker therapy and primary angioplasty: what is the controversy?. J Am Coll Cardiol, 43(10) 1788-1790.
DOI:10.1016/j.jacc.2004.03.001

Fluoroscopy Procedure. (n.d.). Retrieved May 11, 2021, from https://www.hopkinsmedicine.org/health/treatment-tests-and-therapies/fluoroscopy-procedure

Fischman, D.L., Leon, M.B., Baim, D.S., Schatz, R.A., Savage, M.P., Penn, I., Detre, K., Veltri, L., Ricci, D., & Nobuyoshi, M. (1994). A randomized comparison of coronary-stent placement and balloon angioplasty in the treatment of coronary artery disease. Stent Restenosis Study Investigators. *New England Journal of Medicine, 331*(8), 496-501. DOI: 10.1056/NEJM199408253310802

Herrick, J. B. (1912). Clinical features of sudden obstruction of the coronary arteries. *Journal of the American Medical Association, 59*(23), 2015-2022.

Higashida, R. T., Meyers, P. M., Phatouros, C. C., Connors, J. J., Barr, J. D., & Sacks, D. (2004). Reporting Standards for Carotid Artery Angioplasty and Stent Placement. Stroke, 35(5).
DOI: 10.1161/01.str.0000125713.02090.27

Holzapfel, G. A., Schulze-Bauer, C. A., & Stadler, M. (2000). Mechanics of angioplasty: wall, balloon and stent. ASME Applied Mechanics Division-Publications-AMD, 242, 141-156.

Hueb, W.A., Soares, P.R., Oliveira, S.A., Ariê, S., Helena, R., Cardoso, A., Wajsbrot, D.B., Luiz, A., Cesar, M., Jatene, A.D., & Ramires, J.A.F. (1999). *Five-Year Follow-Up of the Medicine, Angioplasty, or Surgery Study. Journal of Circulation, 100*(19), 107-113. DOI: 10.1161/01.cir.100.suppl_2.ii-107

Iqbal, J., Gunn, J., & Serruys, P. W. (2013). Coronary stents: historical development, currentstatus and future directions. *British Medical Bulletin, 106*(1), 193-211. DOI:10.1093/bmb/ldt009

Jaguszewski, M., Ghadri, J. R., Zipponi, M., Bataiosu, D. R., Diekmann, J., Geyer, V., Neumann, C. A., Huber, M. A., Hagl, C., Erne, P., Lüscher, T. F., & Templin, C. (2015). Feasibility of second-generation bioresorbable vascular scaffold implantation in complex anatomical and clinical scenarios. *Clinical Research in Cardiology, 104*(2), 124–135. DOI: 10.1007/s00392-014-0757-4

Janssen, M. Busch, C. Rödiger, M. Hamm,U. (2016). Motives of consumers following a vegan diet and their attitudes towards animal agriculture, Volume 105, Pages 643-651, et al.ISSN 0195-6663,
DOI: 10.1016/j.appet.2016.06.039.

Jeewandara, T. M., Wise, S. G., & Ng, M. K. C. (2014). Biocompatibility of coronary stents. *Materials, 7*(2), 769–786
DOI: 10.3390/ma7020769

Jinnouchi, H., Torii, S., Sakamoto, A., Kolodgie, F. D., Virmani, R., & Finn, A. V. (2019). Fully bioresorbable vascular scaffolds: Lessons learned and future directions. *Nature Reviews Cardiology, 16*(5), 286–304.
DOI: 10.1038/s41569-018-0124-7

Kang, C. H., Yang, S. B., Lee, W. H., Ahn, J. H., Goo, D. E., Han, N. J., & Ohm, J. Y. (2016). Comparison of open-cell stent and closed-cell stent for treatment of central vein

stenosis or occlusion in hemodialysis patients. *Iranian Journal of Radiology*, *13*(4), 37994.
DOI: 10.5812/iranjradiol.37994

Keeley, E. C., Boura, J. A., & Grines, C. L. (2003). Primary angioplasty versus intravenousthrombolytic therapy for acute myocardial infarction: a quantitative review of 23 randomized trials. *The Lancet, 361*(9351), 13-20.
DOI: 10.1016/S0140-6736(03)12113-7

Kidney failure (ESRD) causes, symptoms, & treatments. (2020). American Kidney Fund. https://www.kidneyfund.org/kidney-disease/kidney-failure/

Kim, H., Caulfield, L., Garcia-Larsen, V., Steffen, L., Coresh, J., & Rebholz, C. (2019). Plant-Based Diets Are Associated With a Lower Risk of Incident Cardiovascular Disease, Cardiovascular Disease Mortality, and All-Cause Mortality in a General Population of Middle-Aged Adults. *Journal of the American Heart Association, 8*(16), e012865–e012865.
DOI: 10.1161/JAHA.119.012865

Kondro, W. (2002). Poverty is the main predictor of heart disease, says a Canadian report. *The Lancet (British Edition), 359*(9318), 1679–1679.
DOI: 10.1016/S0140-6736(02)08611-7

Konstantina, A., & Helen, D. (2009). Quality of life after Coronary Intervention. Health Science Journal, 3(2), 66-71.
DOI: 10.1016/j.hjc.2016.05.003

Krajewski, S., Neumann, B., Kurz, J., Perle, N., Avci-Adali, M., Cattaneo, G., & Wendel, H. P. (2015). *Preclinical Evaluation of the Thrombogenicity and Endothelialization of Bare Metal and Surface-Coated Neurovascular Stents, 36*(1), 133–139.
DOI: 10.3174/ajnr.A4109

Levine, G. N., Bates, E. R., Blankenship, J. C., Bailey, S. R., Bittl, J. A., Cercek, B., Chambers, C. E., Ellis, S. G., Guyton, R. A., Hollenberg, S. M., Khot, U. N., Lange, R. A., Mauri, L., Mehran, R., Moussa, I. D., Mukherjee, D., Ting, H. H., O'Gara, P. T., Kushner, F. G., … Zhao, D. X. (2016). 2015 ACC/AHA/SCAI Focused Update on Primary Percutaneous Coronary Intervention for Patients With ST-Elevation Myocardial Infarction: An Update of the 2011 ACCF/AHA/SCAI Guideline for Percutaneous Coronary Intervention and the 2013 ACCF/AHA Guideline for the Management of ST-Elevation Myocardial Infarction: A Report of the American College of Cardiology/American Heart Association Task Force on Clinical Practice Guidelines and the Society for Cardiovascular Angiography and Interventions. *Circulation, 133*(11), 1135–1147.
DOI: 10.1161/CIR.0000000000000336

Liebetrau, C., Wiedenroth, C., Breithecker, A., Haas, M., Kriechbaum, S., Guth, S., Hamm, C., & Mayer, E. (2017). TCT-64 Procedural success of pulmonary balloon angio-

plasty in patients with chronic thromboembolic pulmonary hypertension—a German single-centre, two-year experience. *Journal of the American College of Cardiology, 70*(18S), B27-B28.
DOI:10.1016/j.jacc.2017.09.113

Loffroy, R., Falvo, N., Galland, C., FrEchier, L., Ledan, F., Midulla, M. & Chevallier, O. (2020). Intravascular ultrasound in the endovascular treatment of patients with peripheral arterial disease: Current role and future perspectives. *Frontiers in Cardiovascular Medicine, 7:* 551861.
DOI: 10.3389/fcvm.2020.551861

Mal, N., Vajpeyee, A., Tiwari, S., Bahadur Yadav, L., & Gupta, S. (2020). Angioplasty and Stenting of Intracranial Stenosis. *IP Indian Journal of Neurosciences, 6*(3), 232–235.
DOI: 10.18231/j.ijn.2020.044

McDermott, J. C., & Crummy, A. B. (2008, May 21). *Complications of Angioplasty.* Seminars in Interventional Radiology. https://www.thieme-connect.com/products/ejournals/abstract/10.1055/s-2008-1074750.

Mehran, R., Nikolsky, E., Camenzind, E., Zelizko, M., Kranjec, I., Seabra-Gomes, R., Negoita, M., Slack, S., & Lotan, C. (2005). An Internet-based registry examining the efficacy of heparin coating in patients undergoing coronary stent implantation. *American Heart Journal, 150*(6), 1171–1176.
DOI: 10.1016/j.ahj.2005.01.027

Moer, R., Myreng, Y., Molstad, P., Albertsson, P., Gunnes, P., Lindvall, B., Wiseth, R., Ytre-Arne, K., Kjekshus, J., & Golf, S. (2001). Stenting in small coronary arteries (SISCA) trial: A randomized comparison between balloon angioplasty and the heparin-coated bestent. *Journal of the American College of Cardiology, 38*(6), 1598–1603.
DOI: 10.1016/S0735-1097(01)01602-3

Montemurro, P., Porcnik, A., Hedén, P., & Otte, M. (2015). The influence of social media and easily accessible online information on the aesthetic plastic surgery practice: literature review and our own experience. *Aesthetic plastic surgery, 39*(2), 270-277.
DOI: 10.1007/s00266-015-0454-3

Morrison, H. (1924). Carl Weigert. *Annals of Medical History, 6*(2), 163.

Mwipatayi, B. P., Thomas, S., Wong, J., Temple, S. E. L., Vijayan, V., Jackson, M., & Burrows, S. A. (2011). A comparison of covered vs bare expandable stents for the treatment of aortoiliac occlusive disease. *Journal of Vascular Surgery, 54*(6).
DOI: 10.1016/j.jvs.2011.06.097

Nicholls, M. (2021). Mark Nicholls speaks to Professor Eric Durand and Professor Rémi Sabatier about Europe's first remote robotic-assisted angioplasty procedure. *European Heart Journal.*
DOI: 10.1093/eurheartj/ehab085

Nicholls, M. (2021). The ongoing impact of COVID-19 on cardiovascular care. *European Heart Journal.*
DOI: 10.1093/eurheartj/ehab244

Nihei, T., Yamamoto, Y., Kudo, S., Hanawa, K., Hasebe, Y., Takagi, Y., Minatoya, Y., Sugi, M., & Shimokawa, H. (2017). Impact of the Intracoronary Rendezvous technique on coronary angioplasty for chronic total occlusion. *Cardiovascular intervention and therapeutics,* 32(4), 365–373.
DOI: 10.1007/s12928-0

Oldroyd, K. G. (2017). Complete Immediate Revascularization of the Patient With ST-Segment–Elevation Myocardial Infarction Is the New Standard of Care. *Circulation,* 135(17), 1571-1573.
DOI: 10.1161/CIRCULATIONAHA.117.025265

Olszewski, T. M. (2018). James Herrick (1861–1954): Consultant physician and cardiologist.*Journal of medical biography,* 26(2), 132-136.

Oomman, A., & Ramachandran, P. (2001). Primary angioplasty: the past, the present and the future. *The Journal of the Association of Physicians of India,* 49, 911–915.
DOI: 11837762

Optical Coherence Tomography. (n.d.). Texas Heart Institute. Retrieved May 12, 2021, from https://www.texasheart.org/heart-health/heart-information-center/topics/optical-coherence-tomography/

Overview of Angioplasty Balloon Technology Advances. (2021, March 16). DAIC. https://www.dicardiology.com/article/overview-angioplasty-balloon-technology-advances

Ozaki, Y., Violaris, A. G., & Serruys, P. W. (1996). New stent technologies. *Progress in Cardiovascular Diseases,* 39(2), 129–140.
DOI: 10.1016/S0033-0620(96)80022-3

Palasubramaniam, J., Wang, X., & Peter, K. (2019). Myocardial Infarction—From Atherosclerosis to Thrombosis. *Arteriosclerosis, Thrombosis, and Vascular Biology,* 39(8).
DOI: 10.1161/atvbaha.119.312578

Park, J. H., & Lee, J. H. (2018). Carotid Artery Stenting. Korean Circulation Journal, 48(2), 97.
DOI: 10.4070/kcj.2017.0208

Payne, M. M. (2001). Charles Theodore Dotter: the father of intervention. *Texas Heart InstituteJournal,* 28(1), 28.

Perry, R.A., Seth, A., Singh, A., & Shiu, M.F. (1988). Success and complication rates of coronary angioplasty in patients with and without previous myocardial infarction. *Europe Heart Journal,* 9(1), 37-42.
DOI: 10.1093/ehj/9.1.37

Pijls Nico H.J., Van Gelder Berry, Van der Voort Pepijn, Peels Kathinka, Bracke Frank A.L.E., Bonnier Hans J.R.M., & El Gamal Mamdouh I.H. (1995). Fractional Flow Reserve. *Circulation, 92*(11), 3183–3193.
DOI: 10.1161/01.CIR.92.11.3183

Pocock, S.J., Henderson, R.A., Clayton, T., Lyman, G.H., & Chamberlain, D.A. (2000). Qualit of life after coronary angioplasty or continued medical treatment for angina: three-year follow-up in the RITA-2 trial. *Journal of the American College of Cardiology, 35*(4), 907-14.
DOI: 10.1016/s0735-1097(99)00637-3

Pugsley, M. K., & Tabrizchi, R. (2000). The vascular system. Journal of Pharmacological and Toxicological Methods, 44(2), 333–340.
DOI: 10.1016/s1056-8719(00)00125-8

Rana, J.S., Khan, S.S., Lloyd-Jones, D.M. *et al. (2020).* Changes in Mortality in Top 10 Causes of Death from 2011 to 2018. *J GEN INTERN MED* (2020).
DOI: 10.1007/s11606-020-06070-z

Ridker, P. M. (2002). On evolutionary biology, inflammation, infection, and the causes of atherosclerosis. Volume 105, Issue 1, 1 January 2002, Pages 2-4. American Heart Association.
DOI: 10.1161/circ.105.1.2

Rinfret, S., Grines, C.L., Cosgrove, R.S., Ho, K.K., Cox, D.A., Brodie, B.R., Morice, M.C., Stone, G.W., & Cohen, D.J. (2001). Quality of life after balloon angioplasty or stenting for acute myocardial infarction. *Journal of the American College of Cardiology, 38*(6), 1614-1621.
DOI: 10.1016/s0735-1097(01)01599-6. PMID: 11704371.

Roolvink, V., Hemradj, V.V., Ottervanger, J.P., van't Hof, A.W., Dambrink, J.H.E., Gosselink, A.M., Kedhi, E., Suryapranata, H., & Zwolle Myocardial Infarction Study Group. (2020). Effects of chronic beta-blocker treatment on admission haemodynamics in STEMI patients treated with primary angioplasty. *European Heart Journal: Acute Cardiovascular Care, 9*(5) 462-468.
DOI: 10.1177%2F2048872617754277

Sanborn, T. A. (1988). Laser angioplasty. What has been learned from experimental studies and clinical trials? Circulation, 78(3), 769–774.
DOI: 10.1161/01.cir.78.3.769

Semiz, E., Ermiş, C., Yalçinkaya, S., Sancaktar, O., & Deger, N. (2003). Comparison of initial efficacy and long-term follow-up of heparin-coated Jostent with conventional NIR stent. *Japanese Heart Journal, 44*(6), 889–898.
DOI: 10.1536/jhj.44.889

Serruys, P. W., Emanuelsson, H., van der Giessen, W., Lunn, A. C., Kiemeney, F., Macaya, C., Rutsch, W., Heyndrickx, G., Suryapranata, H., Legrand, V., Goy, J. J., Materne,

P., Bonnier, H., Morice, M. C., Fajadet, J., Belardi, J., Colombo, A., Garcia, E., Ruygrok, P., ... Morel, M. A. (1996). Heparin-coated Palmaz-Schatz stents in human coronary arteries: Early outcome of the Benestent-II pilot study. *Circulation, 93*(3), 412–422. DOI: 10.1161/01.CIR.93.3.412

Sharkawi, T., Cornhill, F., Lafont, A., Sabaria, P., & Vert, M. (2007). Intravascular bioresorbable polymeric stents: A potential alternative to current drug eluting metal stents. *Journal of Pharmaceutical Sciences, 96*(11), 2829–2837. DOI: 10.1002/jps.20957

Shehata, M. M. S., Abdelmalek, W. F., Kamel, A. N., Mohamed, N. M. & Ahmed, A. M. (2020). Evaluation of wound healing after angiosome-directed infrapopliteal endovascular angioplasty in critical limb ischemia. *The Egyptian Journal of Surgery, 39*: 1170-1182. DOI: 10.4103/ejs.ejs_215_20

Sikri, N., & Bardia, A. (2007). A history of streptokinase use in acute myocardial infarction. Texas Heart Institute Journal, 34(3), 318.

Simard, T., Hibbert, B., Ramirez, F. D., Froeschl, M., Chen, Y. X., & O'Brien, E. R. (2014). The Evolution of Coronary Stents: A Brief Review. *Canadian Journal of Cardiology, 30*(1), 35–45. DOI: 10.1016/j.cjca.2013.09.012

Smilowitz, N. R., & Feit, F. (2016). The history of primary angioplasty and stenting for acutemyocardial infarction. *Current cardiology reports, 18*(1), 5.

Smilowitz, N. R., & Weisz, G. (2012). Robotic-assisted angioplasty: current status and future possibilities. *Current cardiology reports, 14*(5), 642–646. DOI: 10.1007/s11886-012-0300-z

Snyder, J., Adams, K., Crooks, V. A., Whitehurst, D., & Vallee, J. (2014). "I knew what was going to happen if I did nothing and so I was going to do something": Faith, hope, and trust in the decisions of Canadians with multiple sclerosis to seek unproven interventions abroad. *BMC Health Services Research, 14*(1), 1-10. DOI: 10.1186/1472-6963-14-445

Sousa, J. E., Costa, M. A., Abizaid, A., Abizaid, A. S., Feres, F., Pinto, I. M., ... & Serruys, P. W. (2001). Lack of neointimal proliferation after implantation of sirolimus-coated stents in human coronary arteries: a quantitative coronary angiography and three-dimensional intravascular ultrasound study. Circulation, 103(2), 192-195.

Spiliopoulos, S., Reppas, L., Palialexis, K. & Brountzos, E. (2019). Below-the-ankle angioplasty. *Vascular & Endovascular Review, 2*(1):6-8. DOI: 10.15420/ver.2018.19.2

Stanek, F. (2019). Laser angioplasty of peripheral arteries: basic principles, current clinical studies, and future directions. Diagnostic and Interventional Radiology, 25(5),

392–397.
DOI: 10.5152/dir.2019.18515

Symptoms and diagnosis of PAD. (2016). American Heart Association. https://www.
heart.org/en/health-topics/peripheral-artery-disease/symptoms-and-diagnosis-of-pad

Tantawy, M. A. (2014). Cobalt chromium stents versus stainless steel stents in diabetic
patients. *The Egyptian Heart Journal, 66*(1), 5–6.
DOI: 10.1016/j.ehj.2013.12.016

Tarantini, G., Razzolini, R., Napodano, M., Bilato, C., Ramondo, A., & Iliceto, S. (2010).
Acceptable reperfusion delay to prefer primary angioplasty over fibrin-specific throm-
bolytic therapy is affected (mainly) by the patient's mortality risk: 1 h does not fit all.
European heart journal, 31(6), 676-683.
DOI: 10.1093/eurheartj/ehp506

Tillett, W. S., & Garner, R. L. (1933). The fibrinolytic activity of hemolytic streptococci.
The *Journal of experimental medicine, 58*(4), 485-502.

Tong, Z., Guo, L., Qi, L., Cui, S., Gao, X., Li, Y., Guo, J. & Gu, Y. (2020). Drug-coated bal-
loon angioplasty and debulking for the treatment of femoropopliteal in-stent restenosis:
A systematic review and meta-analysis. *BioMed Research International, 3076346.*
DOI: 11155/2020/3076346

Tuso, P., Stoll, S. R., & Li, W. W. (2015). A plant-based diet, atherogenesis, and coronary
artery disease prevention. *The Permanente journal, 19*(1), 62–67.
DOI: 10.7812/TPP/14-036

Varenhorst, C., Lindholm, M., Sarno, G., Olivecrona, G., Jensen, U., Nilsson, J., Carls-
son, J., James, S., & Lagerqvist, B. (2018). Stent thrombosis rates the first year and beyond with new- and old-generation drug-eluting stents compared to bare metal stents.
Clinical Research in Cardiology, 107(9), 816–823.
DOI: 10.1007/s00392-018-1252-0

World Health Organization. (2017). Cardiovascular diseases (CVDs). World
Health Organization. https://www.who.int/news-room/fact-sheets/detail/cardio-
vascular-diseases-(cvds)

Wabnitz, A. & Chimowitz, M. (2017). Angioplasty, stenting and other potential treat-
ments of atherosclerotic stenosis of the intracranial arteries: Past, present and future.
Journal of Stroke, 19(3):271-276.
DOI: 10.5853/jos.2017.01837

Waitzman, N., & Smith, K. (1998). Separate but Lethal: The Effects of Economic Segre-
gation on Mortality in Metropolitan America. *The Milbank Quarterly, 76*(3), 341–373.
DOI: 0.1111/1468-0009.00095

Wang, Z.L., Gao, B.L., Li, T.X., Cai, D.Y., Zhu, L.F., Xue, J.Y., Bai, W.X., & Li, Z.S. (2016). Outcomes of middle cerebral artery angioplasty and stenting with Wingspan at a high-volume center. *Neuroradiology, 58*(2), 161-9. DOI: 10.1007/s00234-015- 1611-8.

Watson, T. J., Ong, P. J. L., & Tcheng, J. E. (2018). Primary Angioplasty A Practical Guide. Springer Singapore.

Weigert, C. (1880). Über die pathologischen Gerinnungsvorgänge [About the pathological coagulation processes]. *Archiv für pathologische Anatomie und Physiologie und für klinische Medicin, 79*(1), 87-123.

Whitbeck, M. G., & Applegate, R. J. (2013). Second generation drug-eluting stents: A review of the everolimus-eluting platform. *Clinical Medicine Insights: Cardiology, 7*(1), 115–126. DOI: 10.4137/CMC.S11516

Widimsky, P. (2010). Primary angioplasty vs. thrombolysis: the end of the controversy?. *European Heart Journal, 31*(6), 634–636
DOI: 10.1093/eurheartj/ehp535

Wilson, M.P., Murad, M.H., Krings, T., Pereira, V.M., O'Kelly, C., Rempel, J., Hilditch, C.A., & Brinjikji, W. (2018). Management of tandem occlusions in acute ischemic stroke–intracranial versus extracranial first and extracranial stenting versus angioplasty alone: a systematic review and meta-analysis. *Journal of neurointerventional surgery, 10*(8) 721-728.
DOI: 10.1136/neurintsurg-2017-013707

Wöhrle, J., Al-Khayer, E., Grötzinger, U., Schindler, C., Kochs, M., Hombach, V., & Höher, M. (2001). Comparison of the heparin coated vs the uncoated Jostent® - No influence on restenosis or clinical outcome. *European Heart Journal, 22*(19), 1808–1816.
DOI: 10.1053/euhj.2001.2608

Yamaji, K., Kimura, T., Morimoto, T., Nakagawa, Y., Inoue, K., Kuramitsu, S., Soga, Y., Arita, T., Shirai, S., Ando, K., Kondo, K., Sakai, K., Iwabuchi, M., Yokoi, H., Nosaka, H., & Nobuyoshi, M. (2012). Very Long-Term: 15 to 23 Years Outcomes of Successful Balloon Angioplasty Compared With Bare Metal Coronary Stenting. Journal of the American Heart Association, 2(1).
DOI: 10.1161/JAHA.112.004085

Zamboni, P., Galeotti, R., Menegatti, E., Malagoni, A.M., Tacconi, G., Dall'Ara, S., Bartolomei, I., & Salvi, F. (2009). Chronic cerebrospinal venous insufficiency in patients with multiple sclerosis. Journal of Neurology, Neurosurgery & Psychiatry, 80(4), 392-399.
DOI: 10.1136/jnnp.2008.157164

www.ingramcontent.com/pod-product-compliance
Lightning Source LLC
Chambersburg PA
CBHW021827190326
41518CB00007B/764